PEDIATRIC POPULATION HEALTH

Cognella Series on Pediatric Population Health for Nurses

PEDIATRIC POPULATION HEALTH

A WELLNESS APPROACH

SUSAN WARD
PhD, RN

FRANKIE WARD
MFA, MA, MS

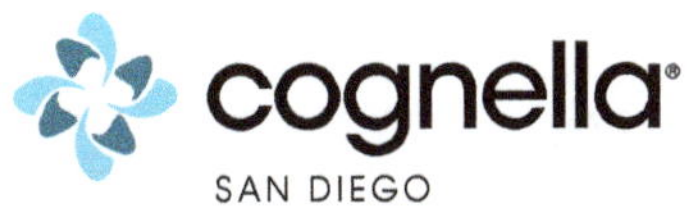

Bassim Hamadeh, CEO and Publisher
Amanda Martin, Publisher
Amy Smith, Senior Project Editor
Abbey Hastings, Production Editor
Emely Villavicencio, Senior Graphic Designer
Kylie Bartolome, Licensing Specialist
Kim Scott, Interior Designer
Natalie Piccotti, Director of Marketing
Kassie Graves, Senior Vice President, Editorial

Printed in the United States of America.

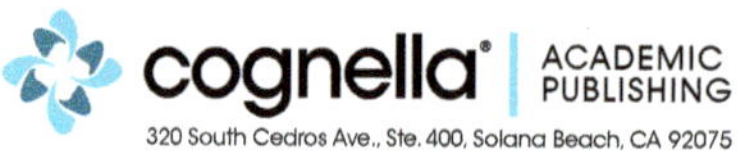

This book is dedicated to Dr. Alice Kindschuh, director of Doctoral Studies at Nebraska Methodist College; Dr. Kiley Petersmith, director of Diversity and Community Engagement at Nebraska Methodist College; and Dr. Meg Blair, nursing faculty member at Nebraska Methodist College.

BRIEF CONTENTS

CONTENTS

ACTIVE LEARNING

This book has interactive activities available to complement your reading.

Your instructor may have customized the selection of activities available for your unique course. Please check with your professor to verify whether your class will access this content through the Cognella Active Learning portal (http://active.cognella.com) or through your home learning management system.

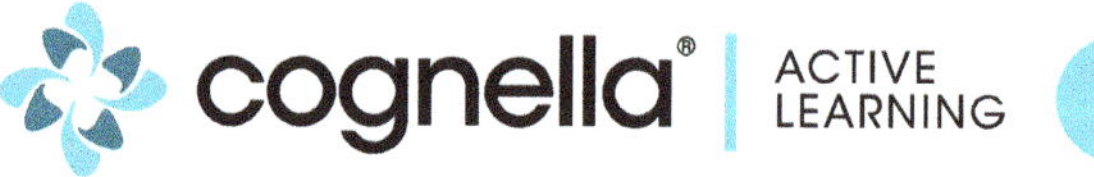

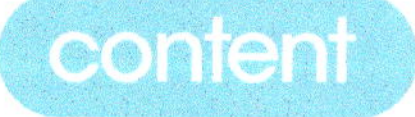

Web-Based Resources: Accessing QR Codes and Links

The author has selected some supporting web-based content for further engagement with the learning material that appears in this text, which can be accessed through QR codes or web links. These codes are intended for use by those who have purchased print copies of the book. You may scan them using a QR code reading app on your cell phone, which will take you to each website. You can also search for the link using a web browser search engine. Readers who have purchased a digital copy of the book can simply click on the hyperlinks beneath each QR code.

Cognella maintains no responsibility for the content nor availability of third-party links. However, Cognella makes every effort to keep its texts current. Broken links may be reported to studentreviews@cognella.com. Please include the book's title, author, and 7-digit SKU reference number (found below the barcode on the back cover of the book) in the body of your message.

Please check with your professor to confirm whether your class will access this content independently or collectively.

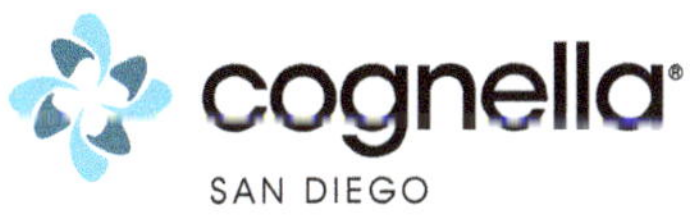

PREFACE

Pediatric Population Health: A Wellness Approach is an investigation of population health, a wellness approach across childhood. QR codes and reputable websites provide a unique means to cover a vast amount of relevant information. The text is comprised of current resources to widen a reader's understanding of pediatric population health.

This book provides an overview of a population health framework. Population health emphasizes prevention and wellness and the eradication of health disparities based on race, ethnicity, language, income, gender, sexual orientation, and disability. An examination of the social determinants of health highlights how to improve the wellbeing of a population through public policies and interventions that go beyond a traditional health care model. Embedded in the population health philosophy is primary care, wherein health care services become accessible, community-based, person-centered, and achieve better health at lower costs. The information on primary care also incorporates health promotion and disease prevention. This text gives information on public health surveillance aimed at improving health issues of the pediatric population, which has risk factors due to age that increase vulnerability to public health emergencies and infectious disease. Children are a vulnerable population and have been shown through epidemiological studies to have poorer health outcomes and have distinct factors that place them at greater risk of poor health conditions than other groups. Therefore, factors affecting pediatric wellness are provided to substantiate a premise that all children must have a fair opportunity to attain full health potentials and that no child should be disadvantaged from achieving full potential due to social circumstances. The following factors influence children's health statuses:

- culture: racial, ethnic, linguistic, or geographical groups and based in beliefs, values, customs, communication patterns, and ways of thinking
- educational opportunities: schools, childcare settings, and at community events
- economic environment: availability of public transit, accessibility of employment, affordable housing, viable businesses, health care access, and early childhood education programs
- socioeconomic status: income level and living in resource-poor districts, which can lead to significant gaps in childhood enrichment activities and educational opportunities

- environmental justice: fair treatment and protection from environmental health hazards and equal access to healthy places where children live, learn, and play
- inadequate health insurance coverage: roadblock to preventive services for chronic conditions such as diabetes, cancer, and cardiovascular disease

Several resources for the topics in *Pediatric Population Health: A Wellness Approach* provide evidence-based knowledge to facilitate the reader's understanding that creating a healthy, equitable community with collaborative efforts between neighborhoods, health care professionals, financial wellbeing sectors, public health, and community development can positively impact a child's health. Section 1 provides an overview of a population health framework, primary care, public health surveillance, and public health policy. Community-based participatory research, the culture of health, functional medicine in pediatrics, community-based health education, fostering healthy communities, pediatric population vulnerability, and the social determinants of health are discussed. Section 2 will make relevant connections to population health as a framework for understanding children's growth and development. Growth and development across children's lifespan is presented along with a variety of aspects such as vital signs, reflexes, nutrition, temperament, and safety that impact children. Developmental screening and standard developmental theories are also examined. In section 3, a deeper dive into exploring the intricacies of a population health framework, levels of prevention and health promotion with guidance in finding accompanying resources and mental health in the context of pediatric care is presented. Additionally, legislation and law that play a crucial role in shaping policies and regulations that directly impact population health are offered. A glossary, reference list, and index follow. Section 4, found on Cognella Active Learning has interactive exercises, case studies, critical thinking exercises, NCLEX next generation style questions, and math questions. It is our hope that *Pediatric Population Health: A Wellness Approach* will help readers understand why population health is a strong framework for a wellness approach for the care of children.

ACKNOWLEDGMENTS

We would like to acknowledge the graduate and undergraduate nursing faculty at Nebraska Methodist College who educate current and future registered nurses (RNs) and doctors of nursing practice (DNPs) about population health. Their educational work creates a more equitable health system that helps individuals and communities obtain opportunities to reach their full health potential regardless of social circumstances.

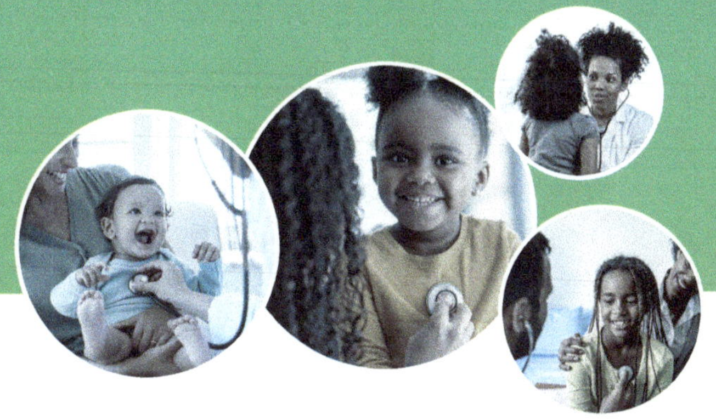

SECTION 1

Introduction to Population Health as a Framework for Wellness in Children

Dr. Alice Kindschuh, Dr. Kiley Petersmith,
and Frankie Ward, Editorial Assistant

Introduction

The field of pediatric population health has emerged as an important area of inquiry and action in the realm of children's healthcare. The health and well-being of children represent a foundational concern for communities as the early years of life are formative in shaping not only an individual's health but also future outcomes. Pediatric population health encompasses a multifaceted framework that delves into the physical, mental, and social dimensions of health in children (Schickedanz & Halfon, 2020). Investing in the health and wellbeing of children helps ensure a brighter future for these individuals and also yields societal benefits, including increased educational attainment, economic productivity, and overall community prosperity.

The sections in this book investigate population health, a wellness approach across the childhood years. Section objectives guide learners on the essential information that relates to population health. Section 1 provides an overview of a population health framework, primary care, public health surveillance, and public health policy. Community-based participatory

OBJECTIVES

- Discover population health as a framework for wellness in children.
- Discuss primary care as it relates to health promotion.
- Explore public health surveillance and its connection to health-related data.
- Comprehend public health policy with the goal of achieving health equity.
- Uncover a culture of health that is built on sensitivity and respect for cultural differences.
- Discuss functional medicine in pediatrics as it addresses the root causes of disease.
- Investigate how community-based education empowers children and caregivers.
- Study the social determinants of health and its impact on children.

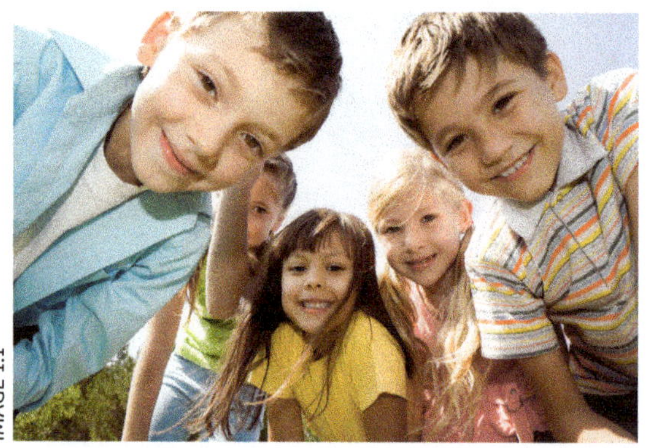
IMAGE 1.1

research, the culture of health, functional medicine in pediatrics, community-based health education, fostering healthy communities, pediatric population vulnerability, and the social determinants of health are discussed. Section 1 also provides the foundational information supporting the material found in the next section. Section 2 makes relevant connections to population health as a framework for understanding children's growth and development and a wellness approach in children's health status. Growth and development across children's lifespan is presented along with a variety of aspects that impact children. Developmental screening and standard developmental theories are also examined. In section 3, a deeper dive into exploring the intricacies of a population health framework, levels of prevention and health promotion along with guidance in finding accompanying resources in the context of pediatric care is presented. Section 4 found on Cognella Active Learning has interactive exercises, case studies, critical thinking exercises, Next Generation NCLEX style questions, and math questions. After reading this book, learners will have a greater understanding of population health and how it is a strong framework for a wellness approach as it relates to the care of children.

Population Health Framework

The Centers for Disease Control and Prevention (CDC, 2020a) views **population health** as an approach that allows health departments to interface with practice that create policy for change to happen locally. This approach uses many partnerships among different sectors of the community such as public health, industry, academia, healthcare, and local government entities. The intent of a population initiative is to achieve positive health outcomes. Kindig & Stoddard, (2003, para. 9) discuss "population health as the health outcomes of a group of individuals, including the distribution of such outcomes within the group." According to the American Association of Colleges of Nursing (AACN, 2021), population health spans the healthcare delivery continuum from public health prevention to disease management of populations and describes collaborative activities with both traditional and nontraditional partnerships from affected communities, the public health industry, academia, healthcare, local government entities, and others for the improvement of equitable population health outcomes (CDC, 2020a; Kindig, 2007; Kindig & Stoddart, 2003; Swartout & Bishop, 2017).

Population Health

Population health refers to the health status and outcomes within a group of people rather than considering the health of an individual. Rather than focusing on the treatment of disease, population health emphasizes prevention and wellness and the eradication of health disparities based on race, ethnicity, language, income, gender, sexual orientation, and disability. The main premise of identifying the social determinants of health (SDOH) is to improve the health of the population through public policies and interventions that go beyond the traditional healthcare model and reach out to the greater community, including a variety of agencies, corporations, schools, and other organization that can promote wellness (New York State Department of Health, n.d.). Social determinants of health affect overall health outcomes and are the conditions in the environments where people are born, live, learn, work, play, and worship that affect a wide range of health, functioning, and quality-of-life outcomes and potential health risks. Navigate to the website to learn more about the SDOH's five domains.

Healthy People 2030

The SDOH are divided into five domains: economic stability, education access and quality, healthcare access and quality, neighborhood and built environment, and social and community context (Office of Disease Prevention and Health Promotion, n.d.-b).

https://health.gov/healthypeople/priority-areas/social-determinants-health

Primary Care

The American Academy of Family Physicians (n.d.) defines **primary care** as healthcare services that are accessible, community-based, person-centered, and achieve better health at lower costs. Primary care incorporates health maintenance and promotion, disease prevention, counseling and patient education, and diagnosis and treatment of both acute and chronic disease and requires collaboration of physicians, nurses, and other health disciplines (American Academy of Family Physicians, n.d.). An integral responsibility of the health professions, especially those in the nursing profession, is to provide optimal care and holistically promote the health and wellbeing of populations. In primary care, nurses work collaboratively in interprofessional and interdependent teams to provide comprehensive care. Pediatric primary care is unique, as it focuses on the family unit in addition to children as patients. This is crucial in a population health framework because children are mostly reliant on others to make decisions about their health and wellbeing.

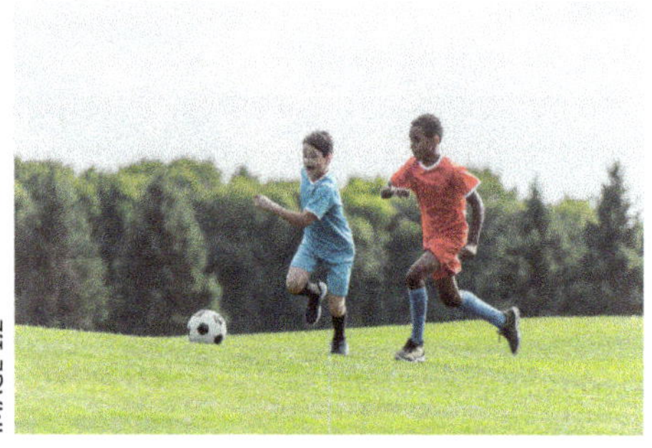
IMAGE 1.2

To support children's health, it is recommended that developmental milestones, growth surveillance, and screening for determinants of health occur at all routine well-child primary care checks throughout childhood. A child's brain doubles in size within the first year of life, reaches 80% development by the age of 3, and is at 90% development by the age of 5. This period of rapid development highlights one age category where rapid growth and change occurs (American Academy of Pediatrics, 2022). The following textbox includes links to websites that provide resources for more information on developmental milestones.

American Academy of Pediatrics

The American Academy of Pediatrics (AAP) website includes Developmental Surveillance and Screening Initiatives pages. These pages provide information and resources to help healthcare professionals be prepared to screen, identify, and care for children with developmental delays.

https://www.aap.org/en/patient-care/developmental-surveillance-and-screening-patient-care/

AAP Parenting

The AAP parenting website has information about children's health issues and resources for parents, families, and caregivers. Developmental age groups are presented with applicable information.

https://www.healthychildren.org/English/health-issues/conditions/developmental-disabilities/Pages/default.aspx

Primary care surveillance is critical to the long-term life of the child to help them reach their full potential. Child visits serve as a method of routine surveillance and monitoring. Iowa's 1st Five Healthy Mental Development Initiative is a national model for ongoing investment in children's mental health. The ethos of the model is that early identification and intervention-based developmental concerns may lead to improved outcomes for children and their families (Iowa Department of Health and Human Services, 2023). Go to Iowa's Department of Health and Human Services website.

Iowa's Department of Health and Human Services

Read about the 1st Five Healthy Mental Development Initiative that serves as a national model for continued investment in children's mental health.

https://idph.iowa.gov/1stfive/professionals

The AAP is a leader in pediatric primary care consisting of pediatricians, pediatric medical subspecialists, and pediatric surgical specialists and is dedicated to the health, safety, and wellbeing of infants, children, and young adults. The AAP (n.d.-b), as part of their Bright Futures initiative, released recommendations for pediatric preventative primary healthcare that include guidelines for assessments, physical examinations, procedures, and anticipatory guidance. This toolkit of recommendations is based on evidence that addresses health promotion in the growing and developing child.

Navigate to the Bright Futures Early Childhood Tools website to access recommendations that exist in a variety of formats, including books, questionnaires, chart templates, and assessment toolkits available for purchase by healthcare professions, insurance companies, or interested community members (American Academy of Pediatrics, n.d.-b).

Bright Futures Early Childhood Tools
Early childhood tools are grouped by visits in English and Spanish.

https://www.aap.org/en/practice-management/bright-futures/bright-futures-materials-and-tools/bright-futures-tool-and-resource-kit/bright-futures-early-childhood-tools/

An example of a major health concern in the United States is children's lead exposure. The contact occurs through touching, swallowing, or breathing in the lead dust. Exposure to lead can seriously affect health, as damage can alter a child's brain and/or nervous system as well as slow growth and development. Children exposed to lead are at higher risk for long-term developmental and health issues.

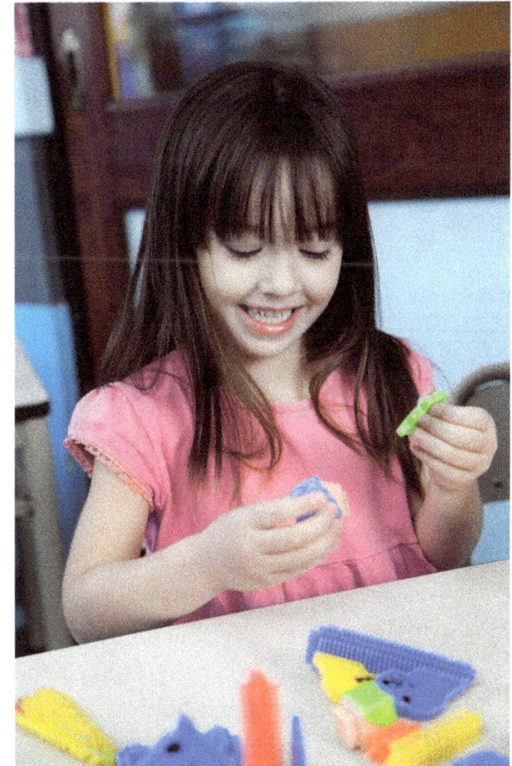

IMAGE 1.3

As a population-based public health issue, the CDC (2022) is committed to diminishing lead poisoning in children by providing blood lead testing, reporting, and surveillance. Families with children who have become exposed to lead can become knowledgeable about childhood lead poisoning, its testing, and treatment measures. The following textbox includes a link to the CDC's Childhood Lead Poisoning Prevention Program website, which includes a wealth of information about this issue.

Diminishing Lead Poisoning in Children

This website is dedicated to reducing childhood lead poisoning.

https://www.cdc.gov/nceh/lead/default.htm

Early Childhood Tools

Be sure to read implementation stories for shared lessons using the Bright Futures Guidelines.

https://brightfutures.aap.org/materials-and-tools/tool-and-resource-kit/Pages/Early-Childhood-Tools.aspx

U.S. Department of Health and Human Services, Health Resources and Services Administration

Learn more about HRSA.

https://www.hrsa.gov/

The AAP website has evidence-based and up-to-date resources to guide professionals in their clinical practice to promote children's health. Included in those resources is in-depth information to review concerns of parents, special healthcare needs, medical problems, and gross and fine motor development.

As mentioned previously, Bright Futures is a national health promotion and prevention initiative led by the AAP and supported, in part, by the Department of Health and Human Services, Health Resources and Services Administration, and the Maternal and Child Health Bureau (MCHB; n.d.-b). The forms on the website relate to preventive health supervision and health screening for infants, children, and adolescents (such as lead exposure discussed previously).

The Bright Futures website also contains a variety of materials and tools, information for health care professionals, promotes health at the state and community levels and provides a framework to partner with professionals about children's health. The following textbox includes a link to Bright Futures.

Because population health focus is on communities, on a national level, the Health Resources and Services Administration as an agency of the U.S. Department of Health and Human Services (HRSA) provides resources for equitable health care to the nation's highest-need communities. These programs support people with low incomes, people with HIV, pregnant people, children, parents, rural communities, transplant patients, and the health workforce. The website in the textbox gives more information on equitable healthcare and reaching those most in need (i.e., underserved populations).

Public Health Surveillance

What is public health surveillance, and why is it important? **Public health surveillance** is the systematic and ongoing collection, analysis, and interpretation of health-related data (CDC, 2018a; Klaucke et al., 1988).

Importance

Public health surveillance eases planning, implementation, and evaluation of public health practice, as well as dissemination of data to aid those responsible for prevention and control (CDC, 2018a; Klaucke et al., 1988). Public health surveillance is important in reducing the threat of infectious and noninfectious diseases potentially changing the health of a population. Surveillance provides an understanding of the health problem to guide public and private health personnel, governmental leaders, and the public on policies and practices aimed at improving health issues (CDC, 2018a).

Factors collected and measured in surveillance, at a minimum, include the number of cases (incidence and prevalence), severity of cases, and mortality rate (Klaucke et al., 1988). Types of surveillance include passive, active, and syndromic (Nsubuga et al., 2006). The most common form of surveillance is passive. Passive surveillance occurs through providers and laboratories reporting cases or diseases to the local or state health departments and in some cases the National Notifiable Diseases Surveillance System (CDC, n.d.-b). Navigate to the National Notifiable Diseases Surveillance System website in the textbox for information about collaboration on disease surveillance.

National Notifiable Diseases Surveillance System
Collaborating on disease surveillance, to keep America healthy, gives information on surveillance, data and statistics and case definitions.

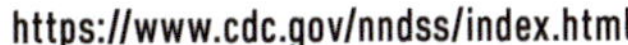

Infectious diseases that may affect a pediatric population (e.g., mumps or rubella) and noninfectious conditions (e.g., childhood lead poisoning) are reportable. Active surveillance occurs when a health department initiates contact with labs or providers and most commonly occurs during a suspected or confirmed outbreak investigation. In the pediatric population, active surveillance may occur during seasonal outbreaks, such as influenza. Additionally, syndromic surveillance is the ongoing systematic collection of clinical data—rather than laboratory data—in real time. Syndromic surveillance is more commonly used where laboratory confirmation of disease is time or cost prohibitive (Nsubuga et al., 2006).

Public Health Surveillance Application to Pediatric Health

The public health system is a primary driver in population health for all, including children. Public health surveillance allows for early detection of and generation of knowledge for health problems and/or changes in health behaviors, expedites understanding of the size and scope of health problems, and measures effectiveness of public health programs and mitigation measures in a public health crisis (CDC, 2018a; Groseclose & Buckeridge, 2017). The pediatric population has age-specific risk factors that increase vulnerability to public health emergencies and infectious disease. Through use of public health surveillance data, the pediatric practitioner in the healthcare or school setting can adapt assessment and screening tools to ensure the early detection of health problems and engage in reducing risk for children.

Public Health Policy

Public health policy plays a crucial role in addressing health equity, which refers to the absence of unfair and avoidable differences in health outcomes among different groups of people. There is a strong connection between public health policy and health equity, as public health policies are designed to promote the wellbeing of entire populations and reduce health disparities. **Health equity** can be defined as providing everyone with a fair opportunity to attain full health potential and ensuring no one is disadvantaged from achieving full potential due to social circumstances (Robert Wood Johnson Foundation, n.d.-a). Striving for the highest possible standard of health for all people and giving special attention to the needs of those at greatest risk of poor health is part of health equity. In other words, health equity benefits all but particularly focuses on underserved communities/individuals who have been or who are disproportionately affected. To achieve health equity, equitable access to healthcare must be present as well as systems to address broader social wellbeing and development.

The Triple Aim of Equity is a framework of addressing healthcare and improving performance of the organization as well as the experience and lives of patients. First introduced in 2008, this framework consisted of three subconcepts, including improved patient experiences, improving population health through better outcomes, and lower healthcare costs. Expanded in 2014 to the Quintuple Aim, this program improves the lives of populations and now includes the addition of the workforce as the fourth concept, addressing burnout among healthcare workers (Cheney, 2022). Go to the website in the textbox for more detailed information on the 4 Quintuple Aim quadrants: improving population health, reducing cost of care, enhancing the patient experience and improving provider satisfaction.

Quadruple Aim

The Quadruple Aim, developed by the Institute for Healthcare Improvement, developed a framework that is now widely accepted by public and private health organizations as a means for optimizing health system performance.

https://www.strategiesforqualitycare.com/quadruple-aim

Health disparities are systemic differences in health outcomes of certain populations because of social determinants. The National Academies of Sciences, Engineering, and Medicine (2019) make a particularly important implication by asserting that health disparities can be affected or potentially eliminated by policy, research, and practice changes across major system structures. Herein lies the importance of public health policy and the implications of addressing root causes of disease in the prevention stage.

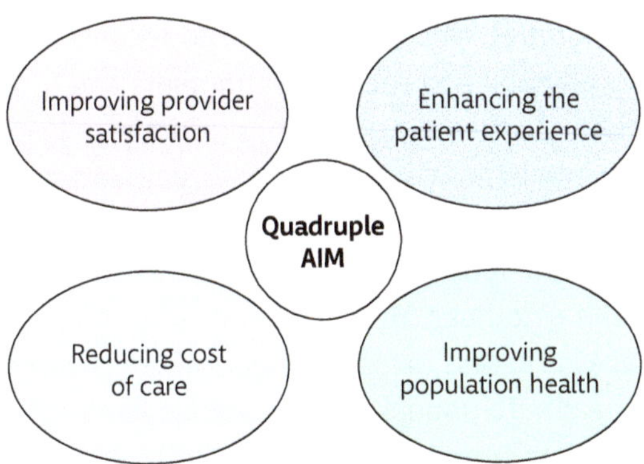

Figure 1.1 Quadruple Aim

In the article provided in the textbox, Bhattacharya and Bhatt (2017), explore seven foundational principles to guide practitioners and policymakers in population health policy that specifically addresses current challenges, including healthcare costs, aging population, shortages in healthcare workforce, and health disparities. These seven principles are in response to the following questions:

1. What is population health policy?
2. What aspects of prevention should population health policy prioritize?
3. How is population health policy developed?
4. Should population health policy be uniform?
5. What standards are used to measure the effectiveness of population health policy?
6. How should we evaluate population health policy?
7. How does population health policy inform population health management?

The following textbox includes a link to an article about the seven foundational principles of population health policy.

Seven Foundational Principles of Population Health Policy

The seven principles of population health policy are written in response to questions posed by both public and private sectors.

https://www.ncbi.nlm.nih.gov/pmc/articles/PMC5649396/

Various experts have referred to health policy efforts as moving to an upstream approach, addressing systems and policies that prevent disease and promote health. Rescuing people downstream is currently a major core function of professional nursing and Western medicine. This means addressing disease after it has occurred, rescuing individuals and communities who are in crisis mode, and focusing on individual behaviors. Addressing physical and social environments and healthcare systems are midstream approaches. Upstream approaches address policies that affect social determinants of health interactions and position systems and structures that promote and maintain health and holistic wellness. In the most basic understanding, no amount of healthcare provided can substitute for meeting basic needs like stable housing and access to food and resources. Health professionals have a basic obligation to address the SDOH because access to food, water, and safe environments/housing are core components to health. To understand the unique needs of populations, healthcare systems must work in proximity to the issues or work with those who have proximity to the issues. Targeted upstream approaches that address key determinants of health, such as where children live, play, and attend school, are important contributors to promote the overall health of populations. The next textbox includes a link to a TED Talk by Rishi Manchanda, who offers a compelling description of this idea of upstream approaches.

Historically, challenges and disadvantages existed when addressing SDOH in policy models. Nationally, poor health outcomes are the result of disparities and

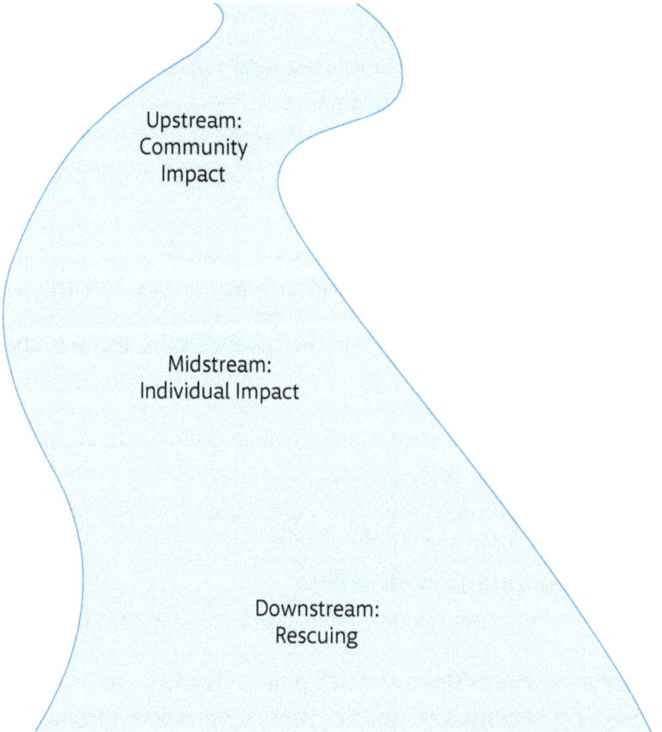

Figure 1.2 Social Determinants and Social Needs: Moving Beyond the Midstream

create financial implications to treat those outcomes across populations. Social justice is essential for ending health disparities. The effects of social factors on health outcomes are often complex and interconnected across many systems, making it hard to find a definitive cause or solution. Building a policy process for a problem with no clear solution poses difficulties in finding support from key stakeholders for lobbying, approval, and dissemination. To positively influence health of populations, U.S. policy leaders need to increase access, create equality in healthcare delivery, and implement more social services support to affect the factors that change health. Despite the expense, Americans underperform on nearly every metric measured. Weinstein et al., (2017) report that the United States actually has worse health outcomes, including higher infant mortality and maternal mortality, higher premature deaths, highest chronic disease and mental illness burden, an obesity rate 2 times higher than other countries, and some of the highest rates of hospitalizations related to chronic disease. The textbox includes a link to a Commonwealth Fund Report by Weinstein et al., (2017).

Ted Talk: *What Makes Us Get Sick? Look Upstream*

An upstream approach used in health care is necessary to meet pediatric population health needs.

https://www.ted.com/talks/rishi_manchanda_what_makes_us_get_sick_look_upstream?utm_campaign=tedspread&utm_medium=referral&utm_source=tedcomshare

U.S. Health Care from a Global Perspective, 2019: Higher Spending, Worse Outcomes?

This report highlights the fact that the United States spends 2 times per capita on healthcare expenses than any other country.

https://www.commonwealthfund.org/publications/issue-briefs/2020/jan/us-health-care-global-perspective-2019

Teitelbaum and Wilensky (2017) point out that the United States is the only developed nation that has not implemented a healthcare insurance system that protects health as a fundamental right. Allowing discrimination to occur based on ability to pay, where individuals live, or on insurance coverage is no longer an acceptable practice. A disparity exists in the United States in terms of health outcomes based on race/ethnicity and/or the zip code of where people live. Across the nation, impoverished populations have higher numbers of people who go hungry, experience food deserts, and crime as well as poorer access to healthcare, primary physicians, quality education, and job opportunities. Millions of children live in communities lacking in resources such as safe housing, space to play, equitable schools, education opportunities, and access to healthy foods. This situation is a result of systemic failures. Researchers have developed the Child Opportunity Index to aid society leaders to identify and address disparities and build social and physical environments to support the growth and quality of communities. The purpose of the tool is to use

Data for a Diverse and Equitable Future
Explore data using the Child Opportunity Index mapping tool.

https://www.diversitydatakids.org/maps/

maps and charts for a visualization of several indices that measure neighborhood conditions where children need to thrive; including the Overall Child Opportunity Index, Social and Economic Index, Health and Environment Index, and Education Index. The textbox includes a link to the Child Opportunity Index.

To work toward health equity, nurses and other professionals in the healthcare systems should focus on developing skills and experience in leadership, advocacy, research, and policy formation. The American Nurses Association (2016) states the scope of nursing includes involvement in policy, advocacy, and education at the highest levels. Disparities in public health are complex and play a significant role in the health of populations. Read the article found in the textbox for a summary of the approaches and how the work is captured by the National Institute of Minority Health and Health Disparities (NIMHD) as a framework to achieve health equity.

Intervention and Public Policy Pathways to Achieve Health Care Equity
The following resource highlights important policy and system structure pathways to achieve healthcare equity.

https://www.ncbi.nlm.nih.gov/pmc/articles/PMC6679008/

Community-based Participatory Research

Community-based participatory research acknowledges community as a unit and builds on the strengths and resources existing within the community. This research builds a relationship and partnership that is collaborative and equitable. This mutually beneficial relationship fosters co-learning and ability-building while shaping the knowledge of the community. It is critically important that partnerships are built on a solid foundation of trust and rapport, recognizing the unique cultural factors that influence the community and thus influence the interactions within the partnership as well as understanding the needs of the community and intentionally using the community strengths to address those needs. There is power in organizing and power in awareness; promoting health equity works best with community partners who are on the ground and close to the issues that need addressing. The American Association of Colleges of Nursing (n.d.) has guiding principles and implementation toolkits available to help academic institutions create effective partnerships. The next textbox includes a link to the guiding principles for academic-practice partnerships.

Guiding Principles for Academic-Practice Partnerships
Find information on guiding principles, expectations and outcome matrix, award opportunities, implementation tool kit, exemplars and webinars.

https://www.aacnnursing.org/our-initiatives/education-practice/academic-practice-partnerships/the-guiding-principles-for-academic-practice-partnerships

Collaboration of stakeholders in addressing population health is helpful. This involves using each other's strengths and resources to address community needs while maximizing efforts through a diverse and collective method. Bringing together stakeholders from diverse backgrounds with different talents can also create challenges (National Academy of Sciences, Engineering, and Medicine et al., 2017). The focus of collaborative efforts should be on a shared vision and value system that emphasizes the health outcome goals of the stakeholders. Human-centered design is an approach to address health equity that puts the community at the center of outcome. Working across sectors in multi-collaborative partnerships creates avenues to address various SDOH (National Academies of Sciences, Engineering, and Medicine et al., 2017). Leaning into the community through a mutually beneficial relationship creates an opportunity to not only gain trust and rapport with community individuals to understand their needs but also use strengths and assets to work collaboratively to address gaps in healthcare services. Being interested in people's priorities, values, challenges, and issues creates a committed mindset to solve problems. Healthcare professionals, including nurses, around the United States are working to change communities one step at a time. Partnering with other entities helps open doors and supports these courageous efforts. At the heart of this work is the engagement in relationships and alignment of action to create more equitable affiliations.

The American Association of Colleges (n.d.) of Nursing Practice Partnerships Tool Kit "facilitates the development, growth, and evaluation of academic-practice partnerships as a fundamental condition to advance nursing practice and improve the quality of care and enhance patient outcomes" (para. 1). The textbox includes a link to Academic-Practice Partnership Resources.

Academic-Practice Partners Implementation Tool Kit

In this tool kit discover strategies on how to begin and sustain academic-practice partnerships.

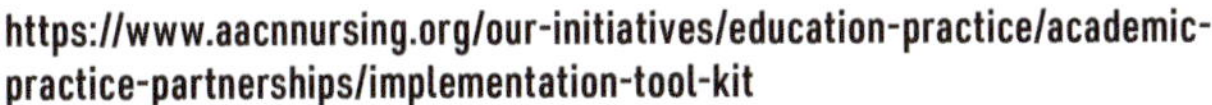

https://www.aacnnursing.org/our-initiatives/education-practice/academic-practice-partnerships/implementation-tool-kit

The National Academies of Sciences, Engineering, and Medicine website includes a link to their 2019 book *Achieving Behavioral Health Equity for Children, Families and Communities.* The book covers the proceedings of a workshop they held in November 2017 to promote children's cognitive, affective, and behavioral health. The workshop focused on a children's socioecological developmental model "to explore health equity of children and families, including those with complex needs and chronic conditions" (The National Academies of Sciences, Engineering, and Medicine, 2019, p. 89). The textbox includes a link to National Academies of Sciences, Engineering, and Medicine.

National Academies of Sciences, Engineering, and Medicine

If interested in purchasing the book or signing-up for a free pdf download navigate to this website.

https://nap.nationalacademies.org/catalog/25347/achieving-behavioral-health-equity-for-children-families-and-communities-proceedings

The National Academies Press also published *Communities in Action: Pathways to Health Equity*, which has a broad array of information and resources related to health equity. To learn more about collaboration of stakeholders and review recommendations on various sectors' participation in collaborative efforts, review the following resource:

The National Academies Press
Learn about communities in action pathways to health equity.
https://www.ncbi.nlm.nih.gov/books/NBK425848/pdf/Bookshelf_NBK425848.pdf

A Culture of Health

A culture of health and a population health framework are interconnected concepts in public health that focus on improving the health and wellbeing of communities and populations. **Culture** refers to group membership based on racial, ethnic, linguistic, or geographical groups but it also refers to a collection of beliefs, values, customs, communication patterns, and ways of thinking (CDC, 2022a). Culture fosters a sense of wellbeing (mental, psychological, spiritual, social, and emotional health; Thomas & Fiote, 2020). A culture of health is a concept developed by the Robert Wood Johnson Foundation (RWJF), a prominent philanthropic organization dedicated to improving health and healthcare in the United States. It represents a vision for a society in which health and wellbeing are valued and promoted as shared priorities at all levels of society, and where individuals and communities have the resources and opportunities to make healthy choices (Robert Wood Johnson Foundation. n.d.-c; Robert Wood Johnson Foundation, 2018). It is paramount to stay abreast of health and health care surrounding diversity in the United States.

Racial and ethnic diversity continues to increase across the United States. The U.S. Census Bureau has a Diversity Index, measured as a percentage that shows the probability that two people chosen at random will be from different racial or ethnic groups. The Diversity Index is updated every 10 years based on census data. In 2010, the U.S. Diversity Index was 54.9%; the 2020 Diversity Index was 61.1% (U.S. Census Bureau, 2021). The website, in the textbox, has information about racial and ethnic diversity in the United States: 2010 Census and 2020 Census data.

U.S. Diversity Index
Diversity statistics, related information and America stories are presented here:

https://www.census.gov/library/visualizations/interactive/racial-and-ethnic-diversity-in-the-united-states-2010-and-2020-census.html

To inspire a culture of health mindset, understanding the foundational concept of cultural sensitivity is essential. To be culturally sensitive, an individual must adapt practices to address health in a way that is culturally appropriate. Lack of cultural sensitivity contributes to inequities in health. Interpretations shape the cultural context of provider interventions (Thomas & Fietje, 2020). The culture shapes the stories of a population. **Cultural sensitivity** allows healthcare providers to understand the society in which an individual or population dwells. Culturally sensitive interventions help build community health and resilience (Girod et al., 2021).

A principal part of creating opportunities for health and wellbeing consists of achieving health equity by addressing barriers listed in the SDOH. The culture of health is a national framework developed by the Robert Wood Johnson Foundation (n.d.-a) that aims to create opportunities for health and wellbeing for all individuals, communities, and populations. The framework consists of 10 principles and four key action areas: making health a shared value, fostering cross-sector collaboration, creating healthier, more equitable communities, and strengthening integration of health services and systems (Robert Wood Johnson Foundation, n.d.-c).

Box 1.1 10 Principles for a Culture of Health

- Good health flourishes across geographic, demographic, and social sectors.
- Our entire society values attaining the best health.
- Individuals and families have the means and the opportunity to make choices that lead to the healthiest lives possible.
- Business, government, individuals, and organizations work together to build healthy communities and lifestyles.
- No one is excluded.
- Everyone has access to affordable, quality healthcare because it is essential to maintain or reclaim health.
- Healthcare is efficient and equitable.
- The economy is less burdened by excessive and unwarranted healthcare spending.
- Keeping everyone healthy guides public and private decision making.
- Americans understand that we are all in this together.

Source: (2015). American Journal of Public Health, 105(Suppl. 2)

Each of the Robert Wood Johnson Foundation's action areas are broken down into measurable outcomes. Making health a shared value means prioritizing health in conversations, promoting health policies, and creating an understanding of how our environment, social relationships, and sense of safety affect our overall health as a community. Additionally, civic engagement, social connections, and being involved in the community creates a sense of belonging, connectedness, and trust and is shown in research to improve health (Robert Wood Johnson Foundation, 2018). Fostering cross-sector collaboration means increasing the number, quality, and sustainability of community partnerships as well as policies that promote collaboration among various organizations. Creating healthier and more equitable communities is measured by creating safe physical, social, and economic opportunities in neighborhoods through policies that uplift physical environments, support quality educational opportunities, and implement safety, exercise, and nutrition programs. Additionally, integration of health services and systems is measured by understanding access to quality comprehensive primary care services, collaboration among various health sectors, including private and public health as well as social services, and proving consumer-driven care, where the experience of the community drives the health system.

The overall outcome of the Robert Wood Johnson Foundation (2018) report is to improve population health, wellbeing, and equity. There are several outcomes that are measured: individual wellbeing, managing chronic disease, and reducing healthcare costs. Individual wellbeing encompasses access to and fulfillment of basic needs like housing, employment, income, safety, and life satisfaction. Additionally, reduction in chronic diseases could significantly improve health outcomes among vulnerable populations and is a measure of assessing individual and community wellbeing. Managing chronic disease is achieved by measuring adverse childhood experiences, which are associated with mental illness, chronic health conditions, and premature death. In 2018, 42% of children in the United States had experienced one or more adverse childhood experiences; these rates can be improved by providing better physical, emotional, and social environments in which children can grow (Robert Wood Johnson Foundation, n.d.-a). One important indicator to measure is disability-adjusted life years related to chronic illness. More Americans today than ever before are living with one or more chronic illnesses. In a 2019 report from the Global Burden of Disease study, the total number of disability-adjusted life years for the top 10 chronic diseases in the United States was 34,252,698 diseases (Robert Wood Johnson Foundation, n.d.-a). The World Health Organization (WHO) website, found in the textbox, provides several resources and ways to explore world of health data, for instance air pollution, environmental health, assistive technology, health workforce and much more.

> The Global Health Observatory
>
> The Global Health Observatory explores a world of health data.
>
> 
>
> **https://www.who.int/data/gho**

When comparing U.S. healthcare system costs to other developed countries and associated healthcare outcomes, the differences are striking. Studies over the last 10–15 years indicate that wasted spending accounts for approximately 25%–30% of the United States' healthcare costs ($760–$935 billion). Wasting spending includes unnecessary treatment, overtreatment, or overpayment (Shrank et al., 2019). The United States as a population spends more on healthcare—over $3 trillion annually—than any other developed country while having the worst health

Building a Culture of Health
Learn more about a culture of health.

https://www.ncbi.nlm.nih.gov/pmc/articles/PMC5568157/

outcomes and highest disease burden (Robert Wood Johnson Foundation, n.d.-a). The burden of higher chronic disease rates is not the only disproportionate burden placed on vulnerable populations. A disproportionate burden compared to income is placed on low-income communities, who spend a larger percentage of their relative income on healthcare than those with higher incomes (Robert Wood Johnson Foundation, n.d.-a). Preventable hospitalization rates, end-of-life expenditures, and falling behind in implementing preventive care services contributes to the increased costs. Additionally, the physician specialist structure and use of resources worsens the fragmented system that currently focuses on treating the disease or symptom rather than the whole person. Primary care and preventing disease through education, advocacy, and addressing social factors can lead to better health, thereby delivering care in a way that reflects the holistic lens of a nurse. Click into the Building a National Culture of Health article to discover how the Robert Wood Johnson Foundation began its Culture of Health initiative.

Communities from around the world provide lessons on how to build a culture of health. They are using their voices to demand access to clean water and air, safe roads, and healthcare. This worldwide movement is becoming more critical due to a variety of population health hazards, such as the lead-contaminated water crisis of Flint, Michigan; pollution from a variety of trash incinerators in Chester, Pennsylvania; oil pipelines being placed across U.S. Indigenous lands; military pollution in Alaskan waters affecting food and livelihoods; entire communities across the world starving; and populations being displaced due to extreme weather-related events. These are a few examples of issues where entire communities are being affected and creating change through resources.

MeasureUp measures and describes the impact of programs on families and communities based on factors related to health. The website offers examples, tools, and resources such as mapping and measurement tools, a deeper dive, an evidence base, and measurement stories (Build Healthy Places Network, n.d.).

MeasureUp
MeasureUP resources and tools to help gage and describe the impact of programs on families and communities and on factors related to health.

https://www.buildhealthyplaces.org/tools-resources/measure-up/

Moving Forward Together provides an update on building and measuring a culture of health. The culture of health perspective is both a shared personal value as well as a broader community value. Civic engagement, number and quality of partnerships, investments in collaboration, social and economic environment, policy and government, access to care, and reduced healthcare costs are all instrumental in achieving healthier communities.

CULTURE OF HEALTH NATIONAL MEASURES

ACTION AREAS	DRIVERS	MEASURES
1 MAKING HEALTH A SHARED VALUE	MINDSET AND EXPECTATIONS	Recognized influence of physical and social factors on health
		Internet searches for health-promoting information
	SENSE OF COMMUNITY	Community connection
		Valued investment in community health
	CIVIC ENGAGEMENT	Voter participation
		Volunteer participation
2 FOSTERING CROSS-SECTOR COLLABORATION TO IMPROVE WELL-BEING	NUMBER AND QUALITY OF PARTNERSHIPS	Hospital partnerships
		Youth exposure to advertising for unhealthy foods
	INVESTMENT IN CROSS-SECTOR COLLABORATION	Business leadership in health
		Federal investment in Health in All Policies (HiAP)
	POLICIES THAT SUPPORT COLLABORATION	Support for working families (FMLA)
		Collaboration among communities and law enforcement
3 CREATING HEALTHIER, MORE EQUITABLE COMMUNITIES	BUILT ENVIRONMENT AND PHYSICAL CONDITIONS	New Measure: Walkability
		Public libraries
		Youth safety
	SOCIAL AND ECONOMIC ENVIRONMENT	Housing affordability
		Residential segregation
		Enrollment in early childhood education
	POLICY AND GOVERNANCE	Climate adaptation and mitigation
		Air quality
4 STRENGTHENING INTEGRATION OF HEALTH SERVICES AND SYSTEMS	ACCESS TO CARE	Access to comprehensive public health services
		Health insurance coverage
		Access to alcohol, substance use, or mental health treatment
		Routine dental care
	CONSUMER EXPERIENCE	Consumer experience with care
		Population-based alternative payment models
	BALANCE AND INTEGRATION	Electronic medical record linkages
		Full scope of practice for nurse practitioners

OUTCOME	OUTCOME AREAS	MEASURES
IMPROVED POPULATION HEALTH, WELL-BEING, AND EQUITY	ENHANCED INDIVIDUAL AND COMMUNITY WELL-BEING	Individual wellbeing
		New Measure: Incarceration
	MANAGED CHRONIC DISEASE AND REDUCED TOXIC STRESS	Adverse childhood experiences
		Disability-adjusted life years related to chronic disease
	REDUCED HEALTH CARE COSTS	End-of-life care expenditures
		Preventable hospitalizations
		Family health care costs

Figure 1.3a Culture of Health National Measures

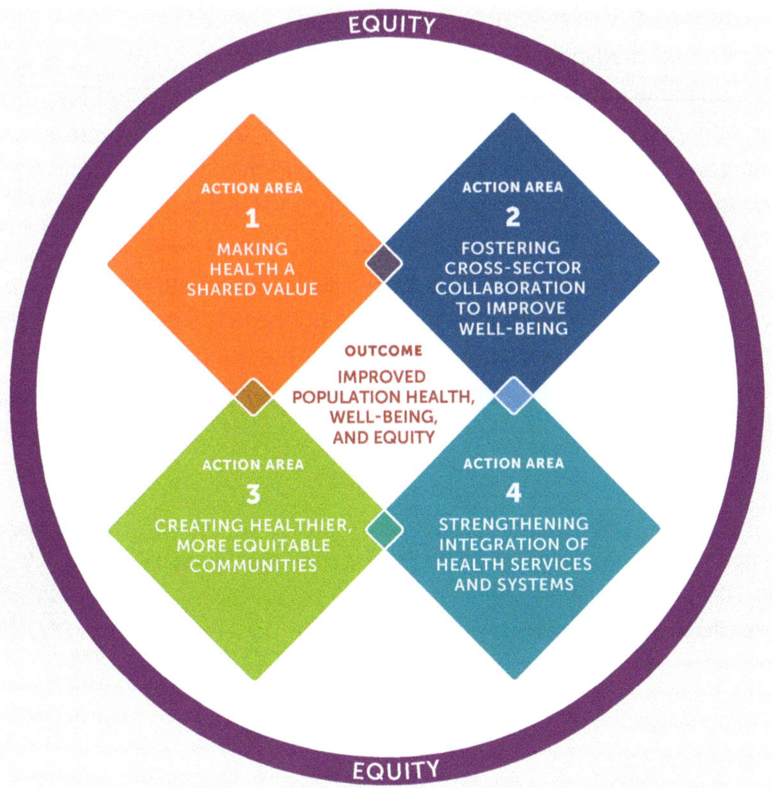

Figure 1.3b Robert Wood Johnson Foundation: Moving Forward Together

County Health Rankings and Roadmaps

County Health Ranking and Roadmaps for Action presents information on building a culture of health, county by county. How healthy is your community? Use the search engine by state, county, or zip code to learn more about health outcomes, factors, demographics, and view a county snapshot. Access the website to gain information about cultivating infrastructure and civic participation for healthier communities.

County Health Rankings and Roadmaps

The 2023 County Health Ranking National findings report examines how well-resourced civic infrastructure gives the space and opportunities to work together and how civic participation helps build power to improve health.

https://www.countyhealthrankings.org/

Functional Medicine in Pediatrics

The underlying factors of many adult illnesses and health conditions have origins in childhood. One means of health promotion and advancing a culture of health starts in childhood with healthcare professionals' awareness of the basic principles of functional medicine. Functional medicine addresses root causes of disease using an individualized, scientific approach (Institute of Functional Medicine, n.d.). This approach includes an understanding of genetics, biochemical interactions, and lifestyle factors. The underlying etiology of a condition may have many causes, and functional medicine practitioners seek to identify and treat the underlying cause(s) of a health condition using an individualized approach. Awareness of potential underlying causes for adult diseases in pediatric patients is of primary importance for pediatric practitioners, because this understanding has utility in the pediatric population to help detect diseases early on, leading to preventable measures. Access the website in the textbox to read about functional medicine as a catalyst in the transformation of healthcare.

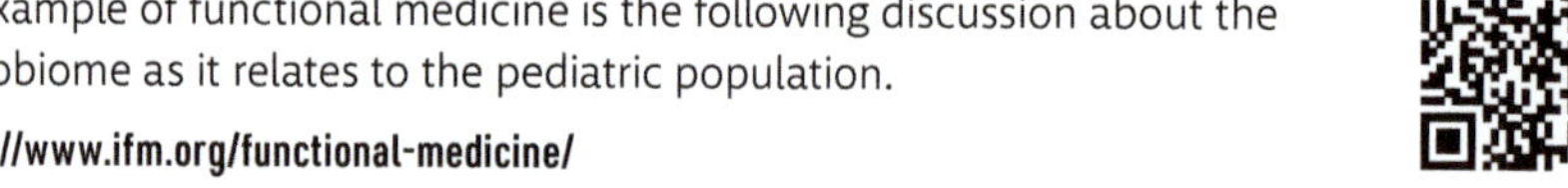

Institute of Functional Medicine
An example of functional medicine is the following discussion about the microbiome as it relates to the pediatric population.
https://www.ifm.org/functional-medicine/

The Microbiome

The **gut microbiome**, a collection of over 10–100 trillion microorganisms in the human gastrointestinal tract, plays an important role in overall health (Valdes et al., 2018). A healthy **gut microbiota** includes high bacterial diversity, fungi, viruses, and other organisms. The gut microbiota is important in metabolism, immune function, cardiovascular, gastrointestinal, and central nervous system health, and mental wellbeing (Shreiner et al., 2016; Sharon et al., 2016).

The Microbiome and Pediatrics

Prenatal and postnatal factors influence a child's microbiome. Prenatal factors include the mother's health, maternal diet, and the health of the mother's gut microbiome (Stiemsma & Michels, 2018). A meta-synthesis by Sharon et al. (2016) revealed that maternal antibiotic use, consumption of a high-fat diet, and maternal stress contributed to fetal dysbiosis, or an imbalanced microbiome. Children born via cesarean section are not exposed to vaginal microbiota that contribute to the diversity of the infant's microbiota. Prophylactic antibiotics during a cesarean section given before cord clamping may further change the infant's gut microbiota. Breastfeeding may mitigate the effect of these cesarean section outcomes (Gaufin et al., 2018; Stiemsma & Michels, 2018).

A critical window of establishing a diverse microbiome is 1–24 months, with the 1–3 months after birth being most impactful (Gaufin et al., 2018; Stiemsma & Michels, 2018). Breastfeeding is of primary importance in infant gut health, and studies also show that breastfeeding can reduce the number of respiratory infections in the first year of life as well as prevent the development of childhood asthma (Gaufin et al., 2016). Unnecessary antibiotic use during the first year of life contributes to **gut dysbiosis** and can have a negative impact on neurocognitive development, leading to behavioral and mood problems (Slykerman et al., 2017). Dysbiosis can also contribute to childhood obesity (Valdes et al., 2018) and to the development of type 1 diabetes (de Goffau et al., 2013).

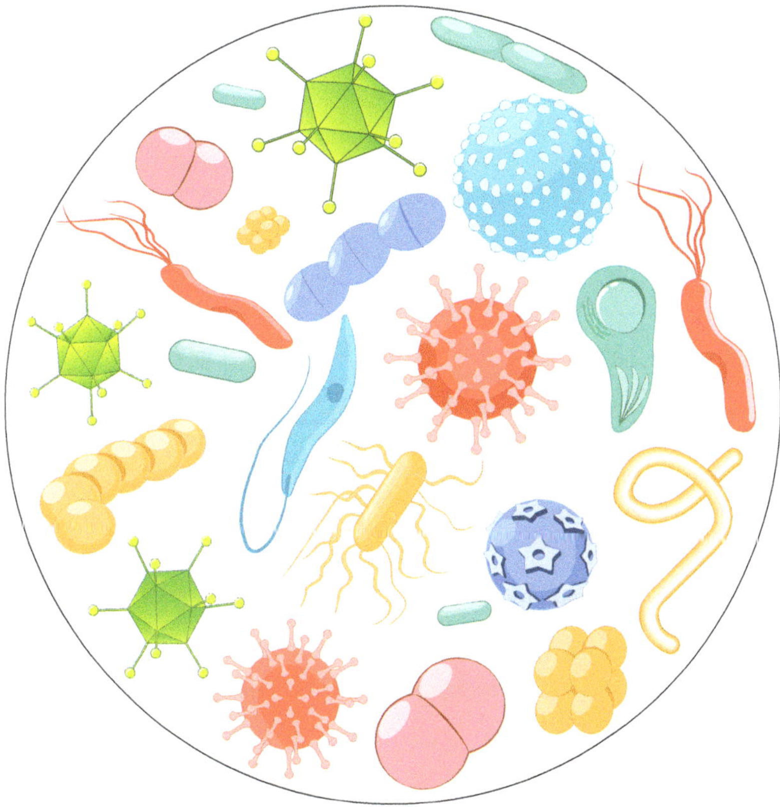

Figure 1.4 Diverse Microbiome

Research

A prospective longitudinal study in Canada followed the children of a cohort of women who gave birth between 2009 and 2012. The CHILD Cohort Study recruited over 2,500 pregnant women. Key discoveries related to childhood health inform the pediatric healthcare workforce regarding key determinants of children's health, including the role of the microbiome. In the textbox, see the website for key research discoveries in children.

CHILD Cohort Study—Key Discoveries

Key discoveries in children include allergies, asthma, obesity, microbiome, breastfeeding, cognitive development/stress, Exposome and Covid-19.

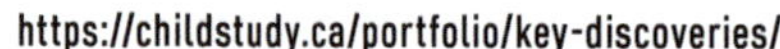
https://childstudy.ca/portfolio/key-discoveries/

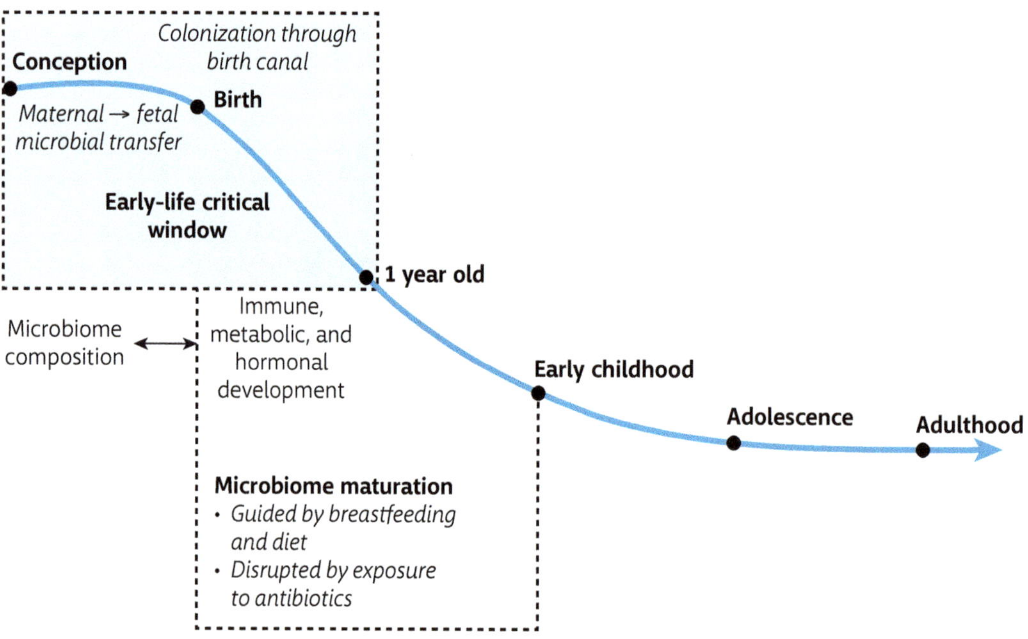

Figure 1.5 The Role of the Microbiome in the Developmental Origins of Health and Disease (Stiemsma & Michels, 2018)

The field of functional medicine is growing, with a plethora of research underway. Prospective longitudinal studies such as the CHILD Cohort Study provide ongoing evidence of the relationship between genetics, epigenetics, and the microbiome for health in the long term. Pediatric healthcare staff have a critical role to play in leading the population to better health now and into the future. Be sure to access the website in the textbox to discover the role of microbiome in children.

The Role of the Microbiome in the Developmental Origins of Health and Disease

The role of the microbiome as it relates to children's health is important information to learn.

https://doi.org/10.1542/peds.2017-2437

Community-based Information

Community-based health education empowers children and caregivers to actively engage in actions that can promote health and wellbeing. Health education should be part of every pediatric visit. Schools, childcare settings, and community events provide community-level opportunities to educate children and families. Collaboration between health professionals and community partners can promote strong population health among children.

The Role of Community Health Workers

Community health workers (CHW) can function as a bridge between healthcare systems and communities, providing a significant role in educating community members and improving health outcomes. CHWs often work in communities where racial, ethnic, or financial disparities exist, thus providing population-based resources to promote health equity. Community health workers are trusted members of, or familiar with, the communities they serve, which positions them to provide culturally appropriate health information and education as well as population health advocacy.

As part of the public health system, CHWs collaborate closely with providers and staff in healthcare systems. CHWs address health promotion and health concerns of children with chronic health conditions. Uchima et al. (2019) conducted a systematic review of research studies involving community health workers and pediatric asthma control that demonstrated the value in terms of asthma-related knowledge, outcomes, and prevention of environmental triggers. Uchima et al. (2019) and colleagues also found that involvement of and education provided by community health workers positively impacted psychological and quality-of-life indicators for children and families.

While few studies are available surrounding the outcomes of CHWs' impact on health promotion specific to the pediatric population, a number of studies exist surrounding the impact of CHWs in prevention globally and in the United States. Heisler et al.'s (2022) study surrounding CHW use and healthcare costs demonstrated those who engaged with CHWs had fewer emergency department visits over a 12-month period. While the cost savings from this was mitigated by an increase in ambulatory care visits, it is clear ambulatory care visits are a more effective and efficient way to address health than emergency department care. CHW programs may also provide an opportunity for education surrounding social outcomes such as community and family violence. Barbero et al. (2022) found that CHWs influenced psychosocial and behavior factors to violence prevention overall. The study by Barbero and colleagues shows the role of CHWs in education and intervention strategies in violence prevention and addressing population health surrounding violence.

Education Resources

Several evidence-based resources are available for children, families, schools, and community members surrounding pediatric health education. Health literacy is a consideration for any education materials. One of the Healthy People 2030 overarching goals is health literacy: "eliminate health disparities, achieve health equity, and attain health literacy to improve the health and wellbeing of all" (Office of Disease Prevention and Health Promotion, n.d.-a, para. 1). Personal factors such as age, culture, language abilities, education, and income can contribute to health literacy. There are several basic factors to consider when creating health education materials, including readability and understandability. The Agency for Healthcare Research and Quality (n.d.) has created a toolkit that health systems should consider when creating educational materials (see the following textbox).

AHRQ's Health Literacy Universal Precautions Toolkit (2nd edition)
The website includes material on health literacy, professional education and training, patient engagement and education and research tools, data and funding.

https://www.ahrq.gov/health-literacy/improve/precautions/tool11.html

In choosing an existing external resource for sharing, it is essential that the information is peer-reviewed and based on the most current research. Educational materials should be readily accessible and provide information that is actionable. One such resource is the American Academy of Pediatrics' comprehensive library of health information ranging from prevention to treatment. In the textbox, access the website to discover expert advice from the American Academy of Pediatrics.

Pediatric Patient Education List from the American Academy of Pediatrics
The pediatric patient education core library is a comprehensive library of trusted health information for parents/patients covering birth through young adulthood from the American Academy of Pediatrics (AAP).

https://publications.aap.org/DocumentLibrary/Solutions/PPE/AAP_PediatricPatientEducation_list.pdf

Fostering Healthy Communities

Community-based education assists in creating healthy, equitable communities that requires a collaborative effort between neighborhoods, healthcare, financial wellbeing sectors, public health, and community development (Public Health Institute, 2020). When done well, this collaboration results in healthy development of children, the ability for older adults to age well, and a sense of connectedness for all residents (Robert Wood Johnson Foundation, 2022). Healthy communities are determined by three main determining factors: built environment, social and economic environment, and policy/governance (Robert Wood Johnson Foundation, 2022; American Planning Association, 2022).

The built environment is the infrastructure of the community. This infrastructure contributes to community residents' sense of safety and willingness to engage in the community. Community walkability promotes physical activity and social engagement contributing to overall health (Robert Wood Johnson Foundation, 2022). Communities that have readily connected to businesses, health-related organizations, and schools foster health and wellbeing. These services might include grocery stores, schools, green spaces (e.g., parks), libraries, community health centers, childcare centers, ambulatory care clinics, and pharmacies.

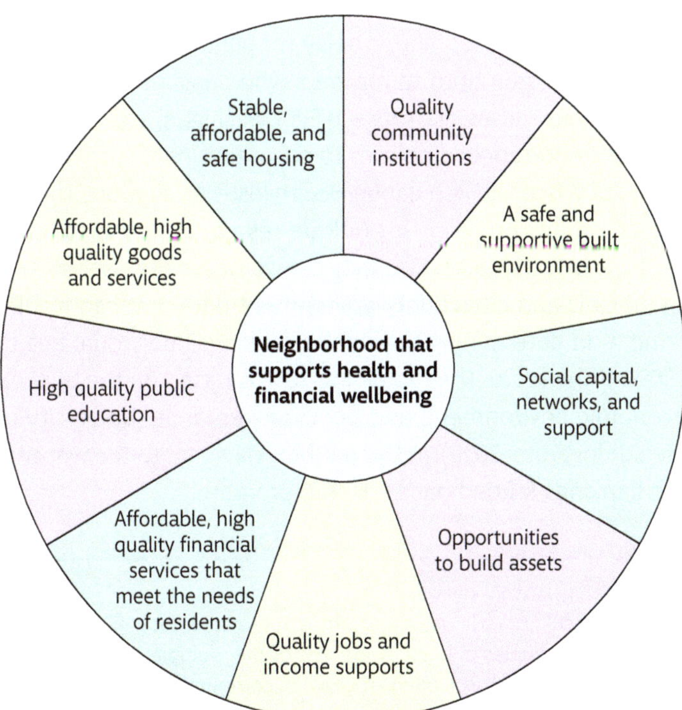

Figure 1.6 Fostering Healthy Neighborhoods (Public Health Institute, 2020)

The social environment can change community and individual health. The social environment encompasses the sociodemographic composition of a community and the relationships among individuals living within the community. Social inequities, including racial segregation and discrimination, have a negative impact on the health of a community. Civic participation and positive social relationship norms have a positive impact on a community's health (Kepper et al., 2019; Robert Wood Johnson Foundation, 2022).

The economic environment includes availability of public transit, accessibility of employment, affordable housing, viable businesses, healthcare access, and early childhood education programs. Individual and community financial wellbeing helps community members in reaching the physical conditions and services needed for better physical and emotional health (Public Health Institute, 2020). The social and economic environment contributes to quality of life and longevity (Public Health Institute, 2020; Robert Wood Johnson Foundation, 2022).

Policy and governance factors have a strong influence on community health. Community and state policies that address air quality and water safety contribute to a community's health, particularly in pediatric populations (Robert Wood Johnson Foundation, 2022). Children are more vulnerable to polluted air due to their smaller, still-developing airways. Policies that address reduction and elimination of vehicle emissions, use of fossil fuel to heat homes, and pollution from factories are necessary to promote community health. Unsafe drinking water that is contaminated with lead or other toxins can cause developmental delays or behavioral health issues in children and birth defects in children born to mothers who consumed contaminated water. Well-known unsafe water crises, like those in Flint, Michigan, and Camp Lejeune, North Carolina, show the importance of policies to ensure residents have safe water.

The University of Wisconsin Population Health Institute supports the County Health Rankings and Roadmaps project. This unique resource measures health in nearly every county in the United States. Counties can compare themselves, thus providing public health officials and city/county government data that can result in community improvement. In determining the health rankings, individual health behaviors encompass 30% of the score. The remaining 70% is based on the built environment, social and economic environment, and policy/governance (University of Wisconsin Population Health Institute, 2022). In the textbox, navigate to the website to discover County Health Rankings & Roadmaps (CHR&R) program.

County Health Rankings and Roadmaps

The County Health Rankings and Roadmaps program provides data, evidence, guidance, and examples to build awareness of the multiple factors that influence health and support leaders in growing community power to improve health equity.

https://www.countyhealthrankings.org/about-us

Pediatric Population Vulnerability

Vulnerable populations have been identified through epidemiological studies as having poorer health outcomes. Example populations include children, those living in poverty or without homes, refugees, people living with disabilities, and those with mental illness. Children are classified as a vulnerable population because they have distinct factors that place them at a greater risk of poor health conditions than other groups. Vulnerable populations are also considered groups and communities at a higher risk for poor health because of the barriers they experience to social, economic, political, and environmental resources, as well as limitations due to illness or disability. Vulnerable populations can be groups that are more at risk due to financial limitations, barriers to education, limited health literacy, language barriers, cognitive impairments, lack of quality, affordable housing, fear or mistrust of health professionals, lack of transportation, or discrimination. Underserved populations receive fewer services, have less access to primary care services, or lack familiarity with health systems. Both vulnerable and underserved populations deserve equal access to and quality of healthcare services.

Age/Developmental Specific Considerations

Children are complex and are more prone to environmental exposures and nutritional deficiencies due to developmental considerations. Developmentally, children start their lives crawling on the ground and even when they can walk, they are closer to the ground. This means they breathe in more environmental contaminants. Infants, especially, learn through oral exploration and can encounter environmental hazards through learning and playing.

Physiologically, children have higher metabolisms, breath faster, have higher skin surface area exposure, and drink more water per surface area, which all increase the environmental exposure through ingestion, inhalation, and dermal exposure routes. Additionally, children are more likely to have nutritional deficiencies due to their fussy eating habits and higher metabolic demands; therefore, food insecurity and access to nutritional foods compound the problem. For example, children are at 4 times greater risk of elevated blood lead levels when their diet is deficient in iron.

Adverse Childhood Experiences

Adverse childhood experiences (ACEs) are potentially traumatic events occurring from birth through age 17. These events may include abuse, neglect, mental illness, bullying, parental substance abuse, parental divorce, death of a parent, and incarceration of a parent, to name a few (CDC, 2021). Community factors such as high unemployment rates, unstable housing, high crime rates, lack of social engagement, and food insecurity may contribute to ACEs (CDC, 2021). These traumatic events can lead to changes in brain development in children, thereby increasing the risk for adverse physical, behavioral, and mental health outcomes during childhood and across the lifespan (Quizhpi et al., 2019). Research indicates that over 50% of children report at least one ACE, with nearly 50% of parents reporting two or more ACEs from their own personal experience (Conn et al., 2018).

ACEs can lead to chronic mental health conditions, such as depression, anxiety, substance abuse, and increased risk for suicide. ACEs can affect long-term physical health, contributing to elevated risk for diabetes and heart disease (Conn et al., 2018). The significance of ACEs accentuates the importance of prevention against and screening children for ACEs at annual visits. Preventive measures can be individual/family or community based. Individual/family-based interventions emphasize the importance of safe, nurturing relationships, positive peer relationships for children and parents, being in a family that addresses conflict positively and engages in fun activities as a family, and having children attend school. Community protective factors include access to medical care, mental health services, stable housing, employment, childcare, quality school systems from preschool through high school, and a sense of connection between community members (CDC, 2021).

Identification of ACEs through screening with tools such as the Pediatric ACEs and Related Life Events Screener (PEARLS) allows for early interventions to minimize the long-term impact. Appropriate interventions may include parental education/training/support and cognitive behavioral training for the child (Pachter et al., 2017). Communities can mitigate the impact of ACEs by having teachers and staff connect with students to serve as positive role models and supportive adults, connecting students to activities that promote self-esteem and peer engagement, and teaching skills for coping and addressing stress. Access the screening tool in the website for more information.

Pediatric ACEs and Related Life Events Screener (PEARLS)

Many families experience stressful life events. Over time these experiences can affect children's health and wellbeing.

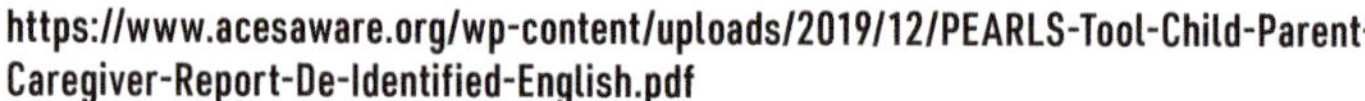

https://www.acesaware.org/wp-content/uploads/2019/12/PEARLS-Tool-Child-Parent-Caregiver-Report-De-Identified-English.pdf

Schools and School Nurses

School nurses are integral to student health and promoting the health of communities. Student health is intricately connected to educational achievement and provides a foundation for future success in adult life. By addressing health barriers to learning and promoting healthy behaviors, school nurses contribute to students' readiness for learning and positively influence school attendance (Johnson, 2017).

The National Association of School Nurses (NASN, 2018) position statement emphasizes the role of school nurses in contributing to healthy communities. It is the position of the NASN that registered professional school nurses should work across sectors, professions, and disciplines to build a culture of health and improve student and community health outcomes by providing leadership, advocacy, care coordination, critical thinking, and mitigation of barriers to health.

School nurses serve as leaders within the school community, spearhead quality-improvement initiatives, coordinate care for students with acute and chronic care needs as well as health promotion interventions, and function as liaisons between the school community and public health systems (NASN, 2018). School nurses hold a unique position in relation to assessing community needs, contributing to plans to address community needs, advocating for children and families, addressing social determinants of health, and evaluating community-based programs (NASN, 2018). The school nurse also collaborates with public health officials in disease surveillance prevention.

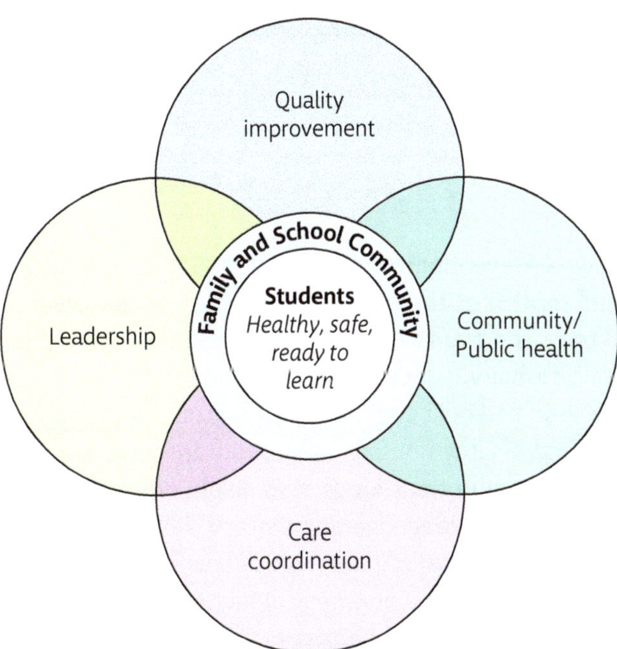

Figure 1.7 School Nurses Serve as Leaders

School nurses are a cost-effective means of providing necessary healthcare to children in an effective and efficient manner. School nurses address health issues that would otherwise fall to parents, teachers, or the healthcare system. The savings in medical care costs and parent and/or teacher productivity emphasize the value of the investment of public money in school nurses (Wang et al., 2014).

Social Determinants of Health

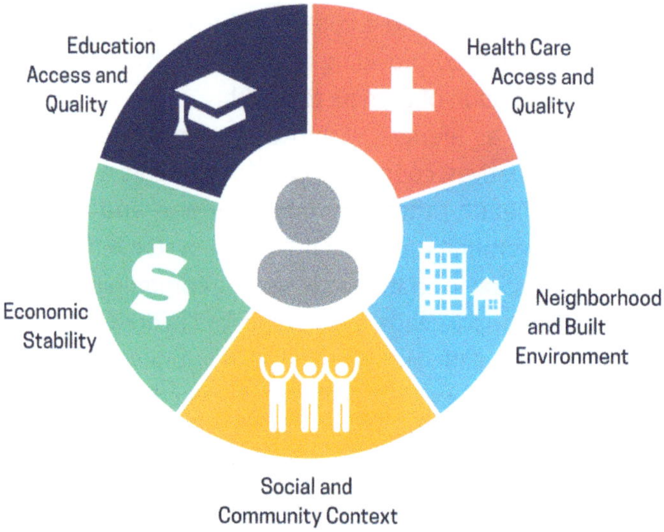

Figure 1.8 Social Determinants of Health

Social Determinants of Health Defined

The Office of Disease Prevention and Health Promotion (n.d.-b) defines social determinants of health (SDOH) as the conditions in which people were born, live, learn, work, play, and pray. The five key domains of the SDOH from Healthy People 2030 include economic stability, education access and quality, healthcare access and quality, neighborhood and built environment, and social and community context. In other words, safe and healthy housing, access to transportation and education, job opportunities, access to nutritious foods, safe neighborhoods, good air quality and water purity, and adequate language and literacy skills all contribute to health of populations. SDOHs have a major impact on people's health, wellbeing, and quality of life and are considered the nonmedical factors that impact health, including knowledge, attitudes, beliefs, and behaviors. SDOH are estimated to account for nearly 80% of health outcomes, both positive and negative, and contribute to wide health disparities and inequities (Office of Disease Prevention and Health Promotion, n.d.-b). Additionally, SDOH are interrelated and compound one another, not only changing individuals and communities but also having consequences for the economy, national security, businesses, and future generations (National Academies of Sciences, Engineering, and Medicine, 2019). Navigate to the website to learn more about the SDOH's five domains.

Exploring Social Determinants of Health

Because children are dependent on adults for their basic needs, the SDOH, as discussed in the textbox apply children's principals to the pediatric population. Income is related to health outcomes in that populations living with higher incomes are associated with lower disease and premature disease rates (National Academies of Sciences, Engineering, and Medicine, 2019). Income affects access to and quality of healthcare. Poverty affects millions of people in the United States and is linked to unhealthy living conditions and increased chronic stress states that influence the affordability of foods, medication, healthcare treatment, healthy housing, and transportation to healthcare (National Academies of Sciences, Engineering, and Medicine, 2019). The prevalence of people living in poverty highlights the need to have health care professionals educated on the health effects of poverty and how to mitigate the problem. Living in poverty exposes children to more violence, housing instability, food instability, discrimination, substance abuse, and incarceration, and they are more susceptible to asthma and respiratory tract infections from hazardous environmental exposure (Francis et al., 2018).

Social Determinants of Health

What are the Social Determinants of Health?

https://health.gov/healthypeople/priority-areas/social-determinants-health

CDC Social Determinants of Health

The Social determinants of health are the nonmedical factors that influence health outcomes.

https://www.cdc.gov/about/sdoh/index.html

Housing

Housing instability is associated with a negative environment, including substandard housing conditions, water leaks, poor ventilation, poor air quality, dirty carpets, mold, and pest infestations. Negative environmental exposures from housing insecurity can contribute to learning difficulties, developmental delays, allergies and asthma, anemia, cancer, or death (Francis et al., 2018). Populations experiencing homelessness have higher rates of alcohol and drug abuse, mental illness, and acute and chronic disease, and they have been reported to have as much as 25–30 years shorter life expectancies (National Healthcare for the Homeless Council, 2019). Affordable housing options provide the ability to meet other essential expenses and create less financial strain. Populations who are struggling to pay rent are going to be less likely to afford utilities and medical expenses.

Food

Access to foods (i.e., food security) has a drastic impact on health and is closely related to income. Poor nutrition is a risk factor for obesity, high blood pressure, diabetes, and cancer. Barriers to, and disparities in, the accessibility and availability of foods that support healthy eating patterns exist and cannot be ignored in understanding how food can positively or negatively affect health. Individuals without a vehicle or access to convenient public transportation or who do not have food venues with healthy choices within walking distance have limited access to foods that support healthy eating patterns. Another barrier to accessibility of healthy food choices is living in a food desert.

In food deserts, food options are limited. This is particularly evident in low-income or rural areas that are likely to have a higher share of convenience stores and small food markets. These options tend to carry foods of lower nutritional quality compared to large chain supermarkets, which may have a wider variety of healthy options. Affordability also influences access to foods that support healthy eating patterns. Low-income groups tend to rely on foods that are cheap and convenient to access but are low in nutrient density. Fresh fruits and vegetables and other healthier items are often more expensive at convenience stores and small food markets than in larger chain supermarkets and grocery stores (The National Academies of Sciences, Engineering, and Medicine, 2021). Food insecurity is identified as a modifiable health-related social need affecting 1 in 5 households with children and resulting in poorer physical and mental health, higher hospitalization rates, and greater risk for health issues like anemia, delayed growth and development, and social and emotional issues (Makelarski et al., 2017). Children are more vulnerable to the negative impact of inadequate nutrition than adults due to growth and development needs. Researchers have found an almost twofold increase in risk of poor health outcomes for food-insecure children; consequently, social determinants like where children live, play, and attend school are important contributors to understanding the prevalence of obesity (Bahadur et al., 2018).

Several national strategies have been proposed to encourage more equitable access to healthy food choices, such as opening supermarkets in under resourced neighborhoods, improving retail access to fruits and vegetables, supporting local farmers, accepting Supplemental Nutrition Assistance Program (SNAP) benefits at farmers markets, and policy development surrounding food nutrition labels and school/workplace food programs. Community-based grassroots work efforts are seen in small local markets popping up in food deserts with increased access and education to develop community gardens or create raised garden beds in homes.

Salud America!

Salud America! is a program associated with the Robert Wood Johnson Foundation that examines peer-reviewed scientific literature on discrimination and bias towards people living in low-income situations with particular emphasis on Latino and immigrant communities. Read the information found in the research review to discover how communities are achieving a cohesive culture for health equity in Latino and all communities!

https://salud-america.org/wp-content/uploads/2020/09/Research-Review-Achieving-a-Cohesive-Culture-for-Health-Equity-in-Latino-and-All-Communities-9-15-20.pdf

The Observer

Click into *The Observer* website to read about profiled Black farmers and advocates, exploring solutions to the issues of hunger and food access in their communities.

https://sacobserver.com/2022/08/rewriting-black-americas-narrative-of-food-insecurity/?emci=c5024490-0735-ed11-ae83-281878b83d8a&emdi=843131e4-2e35-ed11-ae83-281878b83d8a&ceid=5122911

The Federal Farm Bill has been introduced as a food security/food justice and agriculture priority. Navigate to the website to view a panel discussion on food and farm policy with Johns Hopkins Center for a Livable Future and the authors of *The Farm Bill: A Citizen's Guide*.

The Farm Bill: A Citizen's Guide—Panel Discussion (please choose to the skip add)

Food deserts are geographic areas with reduced access to affordable and nutritious food.

https://www.youtube.com/watch?v=9cWOI9z-eZo

The following website considers the accessibility of the food and the size and closeness of food stores to the population. It also considers the quality and type of food available to the population (Coveney & O'Dwyer, 2009).

What are food deserts and why do they exist?

The problem is that not enough is produce but that millions of people can't access it, particularly those who live in areas known as food deserts. Access the website to learn more about food deserts.

https://ffacoalition.org/articles/food-deserts/?emci=c5024490-0735-ed11-ae83-281878b83d8a&emdi=843131e4-2e35-ed11-ae83-281878b83d8a&ceid=5122911

Environment

Geography is an important aspect of environment. Where individuals live matters. For example, zip codes can determine life expectancy. The environment has significant impacts on lives and health; these can consist of schools, homes, soil and water, climate change, and more. The Alliance of Nurses for Healthy Environments (n.d.) lists the top 10 reasons it is important for nurses to understand and be involved in addressing environmental health.

Box 1.2 Top Ten Reasons That Nurses and Environmental Health Go Together

1. Nurses provide healing and safe environments for people.
2. Nurses are trusted sources of information.
3. Nursing is the largest healthcare occupation.
4. Nurses work with persons from a variety of cultures.
5. Nurses affect decisions in their own homes, work settings, and communities.
6. Nurses are trusted sources of information for policymakers.
7. Nurses translate scientific health literature to make it understandable.

8. Nurses with advanced degrees are engaged in research about the environment and health.
9. Health organizations recognize nurses' roles in environmental health.
10. Nursing education and standards of nursing practice require that nurses know how to reduce exposures to environmental health hazards

Source: McDermott-Levy et al. (2022)

Availability of resources in the environment like public or self-transportation, grocery stores, and safe spaces to exercise are all positively correlated to better health outcomes. Environmental hazards such as air pollution, hazardous waste dumping sites and industries, harmful agricultural chemicals, and poor water quality are more likely to exist in low-income communities and those populated by people of color; these communities tend to be more vulnerable to such hazards. Water contamination incidents occur across the nation and world, plaguing low-income areas and communities of color. Navajo nations and Indigenous communities or migrant farm worker communities experience higher rates of waterborne diseases, blood disorders, cancers, and lead poisoning.

Environmental Justice

Environmental justice is the fair treatment and protection from environmental health hazards and equal access to healthy places to live, learn, and work (Environmental Protection Agency, n.d.). The environmental justice movement was created by marginalized groups who seek equality in their communities. Examples of environmental injustice are seen around the globe, including communities in the United States. Access the website to learn more about environmental justice.

Environmental Justice

Environmental justice is the fair treatment and meaningful involvement of all people regardless of race, color, national origin, or income, with respect to the development, implementation, and enforcement of environmental laws, regulations, and policies.

https://www.epa.gov/environmentaljustice

Dr. Robert Bullard, recognized as the "father of environmental justice," is a leading activist in environmental health. Navigate to the website to learn more about Dr. Robert Bullard.

Dr. Robert Bullard

Dr. Robert Bullard has been at the forefront since the 1980s, identifying the causes of and solutions to environmental health issues.

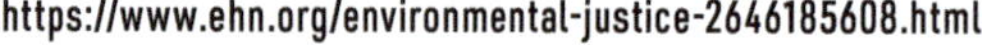

https://www.ehn.org/environmental-justice-2646185608.html

Interested in staying up to date with news and current events surrounding advocacy and policy work in environmental health? Use the website read articles from reputable journalism from around the world, the *Environmental Health Network*, *National Geographic*, and more:

Environmental Health News
Today's Top News.

https://www.ehn.org/environmental-health-and-science-communication-2658582141.html?vgo_ee=YdMxxrHqbf041ccV%2FmDRuovy7T5YEJ8ohjC9vauJg30%3D

Children are affected by a multitude of issues due to their overall dependence on adults. The following is a description of these issues; climate change, racism, employment, health insurance, education, social cohesion and relationships and discrimination.

Climate Change

Climate change, a direct result of environmental pollution, is a complex and ever-growing environmental problem leading to increased incidence of natural disasters, such as floods, hurricanes, tornadoes, fires, winter storms, and drought. These disasters are becoming more prevalent and threatening while straining emergency and healthcare services. Under resourced populations like those who live in flood plains and in housing that is less resilient, such as mobile homes, are more severely affected. Compounding the problem, low-income residents have less capacity and resources to move when such risk arises. Climate change is also leading to heat-related illness, including heat strokes, cardiac stress, asthma, and respiratory disease, due to the increased formation of ozone. Additionally, climate change is leading to more vector-borne and zoonotic diseases, which is causing more foodborne diseases and crop devastation. The increased growth of pests can globally devastate crop growth, worsening the worldwide issues of malnutrition and poverty. Learn about climate change on the Alliance of Nurses for Healthy Environments website:

Climate Change and Health
The Alliance of Nurses for Healthy Environments has partnered with ecoAmerica (eA) and Climate for Health (CfH) in supporting the Nursing Collaborative on Climate Change and Health which aims to bring together nursing organizations to promote nursing leadership in addressing climate change.

https://envirn.org/climate-change/

Racism

Embedded racism in U.S. laws, policies, and institutions creates disadvantage. Black, Hispanic, Indigenous, or other populations of color have higher rates of chronic health conditions, higher mortality rates and incarceration rates, and reduced life expectancies (The National Academies of Sciences, Engineering, and Medicine, 2019). Redlining had and continues to have a significant impact on how race has shaped living environments and income for generations of Black Americans. In the late 1930s, as the nation was just starting to recover from the Great Depression, the New Deal was signed as an initiative to reinvigorate the economy. A significant aspect of the New Deal was to promote home ownership, boosting the economy. Redlining was a racist policy developed to assess risk of who it was safe to loan money to. Race/immigration status as well as environmental hazards were foundational to how this risk was determined. People living within the redlined areas (high-risk areas) were limited in home loans and the ability to build equity and generational wealth. Individuals also fell into predatory banking with high interest rates. Unfortunately, the "red lines" drawn around U.S. cities continue to hold strong, having long-lasting effects on children, families and communities today.

Un-design the Redline

Learn more about redlining.

http://www.designingthewe.com/undesign-the-redline

To better understand racial equity and the public health impacts of racism, the American Public Health Association (n.d.) has delved into this topic, stating, "Racial equity is central to health equity, which is the assurance of the conditions that allow everyone the opportunity to reach their best health" (para. 2).

Racial Equity and Public Health

Racial equity is the condition that will be achieved when racial identity no longer predicts how a person fares in society. To learn more about racial equity and public health, view the following American Public Health Association resource.

https://www.apha.org/-/media/Files/PDF/advocacy/SPEAK/210825_Racial_Equity_Fact_Sheet.ashx

Employment

Multiple aspects of employment, including job security, work environment, financial compensation, and job demands, may affect health of families. Parent(s) employment offers many benefits, such as income, health insurance, and paid parental and sick leave—all which can positively influence health (National Academies of Sciences, Engineering, and Medicine, 2021). Two important benefits of health insurance are access to affordable healthcare and financial protection from unexpected healthcare costs. Paid sick leave allows individuals to seek medical care without losing income. In addition, some employers offer parental leave after the birth of a child. Parental leave has been associated with positive outcomes for both parents and children, including decreased infant mortality rates, improved infant attachment and breastfeeding, and improved access to healthcare visits and immunization administration.

The work environment may create risks for injuries and illness if jobs include repetitive lifting, pulling, or pushing of heavy loads, inadequate quality office equipment, long-term exposure to harmful chemicals such as lead, pesticides, aerosols, and asbestos, or a noisy work environment. Other sources of workplace stress include elevated levels of interpersonal conflict, highly demanding jobs, working evening shifts, working more than 8 hours a day, and having multiple jobs (National Academies of Sciences, Engineering, and Medicine, 2021). The COVID-19 pandemic affected workplace environments, especially jobs that were mandated to be in-person within close working conditions and with limited resources. Certain occupations that were most at risk during the pandemic include healthcare workers, laboratory personnel, morgue workers, and workers whose jobs required close working conditions with limited personal protective equipment (Occupational Safety and Health Administration, n.d.). Additionally, employment-related stressors put people at risk for mortality, depression, and unhealthy coping skills, such as smoking or alcohol abuse. Negative health consequences of unemployment also include anxiety, demoralization, physical pain, and stress-related illnesses such as high blood pressure, stroke, heart attack, heart disease, and arthritis (National Academies of Sciences, Engineering, and Medicine, 2021). Any of these topics may impact children's health and wellbeing.

Health Insurance

Inadequate health insurance coverage is one of the largest barriers to healthcare access. Out-of-pocket medical care costs may lead individuals to forgo or delay needed care. Individuals with lower incomes are often uninsured or underinsured. Individuals without health insurance are less likely to receive preventive services for chronic conditions such as diabetes, cancer, and cardiovascular disease (National Academies of Sciences, Engineering, and Medicine, 2021). Similarly, children without health insurance coverage are less likely to receive appropriate treatment for conditions like asthma or critical preventive services, such as dental care, immunizations, and well-child visits that track developmental milestones.

Education

Education links to disparities in employment because it affects the type of work people do, the working conditions they experience, and the income earned. Higher education helps people secure better paying jobs with fewer safety hazards (National Academies of Sciences, Engineering, and Medicine, 2021). Income from these employment opportunities may improve health by increasing peoples' abilities to accrue material resources, such as higher quality housing and access to insurance/benefits (National Academies of Sciences, Engineering, and Medicine, 2021). Individuals with less education have fewer employment options, which may force them into positions with job insecurity, low wages, and that are more physically demanding or include exposure to toxins (National Academies of Sciences, Engineering, and Medicine, 2021). Education affects the type of employment people have, and the overall income of populations can affect the type of education a person received. Lower income families often live in resource-poor districts; over time this can lead to significant gaps in childhood enrichment activities and educational opportunities (National Academies of Sciences, Engineering, and Medicine, 2021). Adults with lower educational attainment have higher rates of heart and circulatory disease, diabetes, liver disease, and psychological symptoms. Therefore, there is certainly a link between parental education as it relates to children's health status.

Social Cohesion and Relationships

Social cohesion and relationships are important for physical health and psychosocial wellbeing. Relationships build not only a sense of community, a sense of belonging, but also a network of shared resources for the community. For example, stronger connection and relationships to community members provides more opportunities for transportation to medical appointments or childcare centers. More social cohesion is associated with better self-rated health, lower rates of neighborhood violence, and better access to medical care, healthy food options, and places to exercise (National Academies of Sciences, Engineering, and Medicine, 2021). Social institutions like religion and the family are common sources of social networks and social support. In contrast, social isolation is negatively associated to health and increases mortality. Social isolation is a special concern for older adults, individuals in long-term care facilities, or those with conditions that interfere with daily activities. In a population health framework it is important to know about the association involving social cohesion and relationships and wellness in children.

Discrimination

Discrimination is the unjust or prejudicial treatment based on race, religion, age, gender or sexual orientation, disability/ability, and more (Davis, 2020). Discrimination occurs both individually and systemically. Examples of individual discrimination include slurs, micro aggressions, and violence. Systemic discrimination occurs when resources that influence SDOH are differently distributed between groups. Examples of systemic discrimination include incarceration, social immobility, and inadequate quality housing. Redlining, as discussed previously, is an example of housing and economic discrimination based on race.

Sense of Community as a Shared Value
Discrimination: A Social Determinate of Health.

https://www.healthaffairs.org/do/10.1377/forefront.20200220.518458/full/

Discrimination in children, whether based on race, gender, socioeconomic status, or other factors, is a critical concern within a population health framework. Such discrimination not only negatively impacts the immediate wellbeing of affected individuals but also has far-reaching consequences for the overall health of a community or society. The stress and trauma resulting from discrimination can lead to a range of physical and mental health disparities, including increased rates of chronic diseases, mental health disorders, and reduced access to quality healthcare. Addressing discrimination in children is therefore essential for promoting equity and improving the health outcomes of an entire population, as it fosters a healthier, more inclusive environment where all children can thrive and contribute positively to society.

How It All Overlaps and the Vulnerabilities of Children

Predictors of disparity exist in the United States in the fact that health outcomes are based on race or zip code. Those who develop cancer or chronic conditions are disproportionately underserved/marginalized populations who are more likely to have worsened and compounding conditions. As discussed, complex relationships exist between poverty, food and housing security, nutrition, obesity, anemia, and other health concerns. Health disparities associated with SDOH can be identified when looking at health outcomes of morbidity, mortality, life expectancy, and healthcare costs.

SDOH develop a foundation of health early in life; therefore, it is particularly important to consider children due to the foundation of physical, social, and emotional capabilities that develop early in life. Identifying these factors can serve as primary prevention, minimizing disparity and influencing the future health of children into adulthood (Sokol et al., 2019). Approaching primary pediatric care with a population health lens directs providers to screen children in the environment in which they live, learn, and play, ultimately increasing access to medical care for children who may not have access to preventative screening. Research demonstrates the need to understand variables, mechanisms, and causality pathways of nearly 20 socioeconomic or social determinant indicators to address inequalities in health (Shokouh et al., 2016).

For a more thorough understanding of frameworks for social determinants of health and the role of nursing in educating and addressing social determinants, access the following resource.

Frameworks for Social Determinants of Health

The future of nursing 2020–2023: charting a path to achieve health equity.

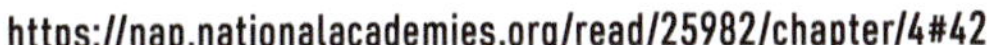

https://nap.nationalacademies.org/read/25982/chapter/4#42

National Center for Health Statistics

In 2022, the National Center for Health Statistics (NCHS) released a report titled "Examining Progress Toward Elimination of Racial and Ethnic Health Disparities for Healthy People 2020 Objectives Using Three Measures of Overall Disparity." This report, in the website, provides the very first end-of-decade assessment of progress in addressing health disparities by race and ethnicity across all Healthy People 2020 objectives. Among the 985 trackable objectives, 33.9% were met or exceeded, 20.8% were improved, 31% had little or no detectable change, and 14.3% became worse.

https://pubmed.ncbi.nlm.nih.gov/36409518/

Box 1.3 End-of-Decade Status of Healthy People 2020 Trackable Objectives by Topic Area

Topic areas where 50% or more of trackable objectives improved, met, or exceeded Healthy People 2020 targets:

- access to health services
- adolescent health
- cancer
- chronic kidney disease
- disability and health
- educational and community-based programs
- environmental health
- genomics
- global health
- health communication and health information technology
- healthcare-associated infections
- heart disease and stroke
- HIV
- immunization and infectious diseases
- maternal, infant, and child health
- medical product safety
- nutrition and weight status
- occupational safety and health
- oral health
- physical activity
- preparedness
- public health infrastructure
- sexually transmitted diseases
- tobacco use
- vision

Topic areas where less than 50% of trackable objectives improved, met, or exceeded Health People 2020 targets:

- arthritis, osteoporosis, and chronic back conditions
- blood disorders and blood safety
- dementias, including Alzheimer's disease
- diabetes
- early and middle childhood
- family planning
- food safety
- hearing and other sensory or communication disorders
- injury and violence prevention
- lesbian, gay, bisexual, and transgender health
- mental health and mental disorders
- older adults
- respiratory diseases
- sleep health
- substance abuse

Source: Office of Disease Prevention and Health Promotion. (2022). Newly released: Vital and health statistics series report on health disparities in healthy people 2020. https://health.gov/news/202211/newly-released-vital-and-health-statistics-series-report-health-disparities-healthy-people-2020?source=govdelivery&utm_medium=email&utm_source=govdelivery

Another overlapping concern impacting vulnerable children is social justice. Social justice is essential for ending health disparities. Lillian Wald was a pioneer in nursing by implementing these concepts and cooperating with social agencies to improve the health of entire neighborhoods (Fee & Bu, 2011). During the nation's greatest economic depressions, Wald provided ice, sterile milk, medications, food, and medical referrals to individuals, families, and neighborhoods; in addition, Wald was able to connect individuals with jobs to earn some income to support their families (Fee & Bu, 2011). Wald emphasized the just and respectful dignity of all humans, poor or wealthy. See the textbox to learn how Wald was a pioneer in the issues of public health, health equity, and educating nurses about the importance that social and environmental factors played in the advancement of health for populations (Fee & Bu, 2011).

Henry Street Settlement, Lillian Wald, an Amazing Nurse!

Founded in 1893 by progressive reformer Lillian Wald, Henry Street Settlement provides social services, arts and health care programs to New Yorkers from 17 sites on Manhattan's Lower East Side. Learn more about Lillian Wald's Henry Street Settlement.

https://www.nyc.gov/site/dhs/about/henry-street-settlement.page

To bring about change to the current healthcare culture, health professionals need a mindset like Lillian Wald's to address more than the physical manifestation of disease. The disparity gaps that communities around the world are facing are widening, which is why the World Health Organization, the Institute of Medicine, and the Future of Nursing Report have a growing focus on SDOH. Implementing a culture of health framework invites healthcare professionals to participate in advocacy, policy creation, research, and the fight for equal access to healthcare and equal opportunities for health literacy and health promotion while working to eliminate disparities.

Identifying the root causes of health problems and providing resources to mitigate the issues before they impact health can be accomplished through assessment tools focused on social determinants of health. Pediatric wellness screenings should (a) be tailored to address commonly identified issues in the community, (b) address serious/fewer common issues, (c) elicit parent perspectives, (d) be appropriate for a child's developmental stage, and (e) be implemented after available resources to address issues (Chung et al., 2016). By increasing SDOH screening, healthcare professionals have an opportunity to gain valuable information on stressors that influence health while mitigating unmet social needs to reduce toxic stress and thereby improve health (Morone, 2017). Opportunities also exist for nurses to develop community-based referral systems and enhance connections within communities (Morone, 2017). Nurses and other healthcare professionals in educational settings may be well-equipped to conduct universal SDOH screenings, as these factors can influence optimal educational development. School nurses also have established rapport and can follow up and advocate for patients. SDOH support could provide children with the health and nutritional support to focus and learn. Schools would better understand the needs of their students and could aid with resources to potentially prevent children from missing school. However, if screening is delayed until school years, it may be too late. Gitterman et al. (2016) highlights early childhood as a key influencer in lifelong health. Access the websites to learn more about the PRAPARE Screening tool and other resources.

Assessment Tools

PRAPARE Screening Tool

The PRAPARE Screening Tool has been translated in over 25 languages to extend accessibility to diverse populations. Access the PRAPARE Screening Tool from the website to understand how the social determinants of health assessment tool has been modified for several culturally diverse populations.

https://prapare.org/the-prapare-screening-tool/

The Centers for Medicare & Medicaid Services (CMS) Center for Medicare and Medicaid Innovation (CMMI) the Accountable Health Communities (AHC) and Health-Related Social Needs (HRSN) Screening Tool is used in the Accountable Health Communities (AHC) Model. Access the Accountable Health Communities Health-Related Social Needs Screening Tool:

Accountable Health Communities Health-Related Social Needs Screening Tool

What is the Accountable Health Communities (AHC) Health-Related Social Needs (HRSN) Screening Tool?

https://innovation.cms.gov/files/worksheets/ahcm-screeningtool.pdf

An Integrative Review of Social Determinants of Health Assessment and Screening Tools Used in Pediatrics

The following article provides a review of SDOH assessment and screening tools used in pediatrics. "Thirteen articles relevant to the assessment of SDOH domains were evaluated. Majority of studies were limited in both the number of SDOH domains screened and the depth of screening. Tools were heterogeneous in methods used to assess SDOH risks and few were validated. Limited number of studies included youth or families in the initial development of tools" (Morone, 2017, para 1).

https://doi.org/10.1016/j.pedn.2017.08.022

The Centers for Disease Control and Prevention (CDC) is a leading public health agency in the United States, operating under the U.S. Department of Health and Human Services. The CDC is dedicated to protecting public health and safety by preventing and controlling diseases, injuries, and other health threats. The CDC, (2022-d) has put together a list of resources to help guide practitioners to addressing social determinants of health. Navigate to the website:

What are the Social Determinants of Health?

Continue to learn about the SDOH.

https://www.cdc.gov/socialdeterminants/tools/index.htm

The American Academy of Pediatrics (AAP) is a professional organization of pediatricians in the United States. Founded in 1930, the AAP is dedicated to promoting the health and wellbeing of children and adolescents. It serves as a leading authority on pediatric healthcare and child development, providing guidance, resources, and advocacy on a wide range of issues related to children's health. The AAP has a similar comprehensive list of resources to guide practitioners in pediatric-specific SDOH screening and psychosocial concerns.

Social Determinants of Health Screening Resources

Browse the resources on this page for information and tools on screening, referral, and follow-up for social determinants of health and managing psychosocial concerns.

https://www.aap.org/en/patient-care/screening-technical-assistance-and-resource-center/screening-resource-library/social-determinants-of-health/?page=1&sortDirection=1&sortField=Year

"Healthy People" is a nationwide initiative in the United States developed by the U.S. Department of Health and Human Services (HHS). It sets specific, science-based objectives and targets for improving public health and reducing health disparities over a 10-year period. Through programs, policies, and interventions, Healthy People 2023 is working hard to improve the conditions in people's environments. This work helps reduce health disparities and improve health and wellbeing for all people. Review what communities around the United States are doing to focus on SDOH through programming and policies interventions:

Healthy People Partners and SDOH

Healthy People 2030 has an increased focus on the social determinants of health.

https://health.gov/healthypeople/priority-areas/social-determinants-health/healthy-people-partners-and-sdoh

Nurse advocacy is a concept and practice that underscores the critical role of nurses in advocating for policies and initiatives that prioritize health and wellbeing across all sectors of society. This approach recognizes that health is influenced by various factors beyond healthcare, including education, transportation, housing, and more. Nurses, as frontline healthcare professionals, are well-positioned to advocate for policies that promote a holistic view of health, emphasizing prevention and addressing the social determinants of health.

To learn more about policy advocacy and committed resources essential to addressing social factors that shape population health read the following article to learn how nurses can be advocates by adopting a health mindset when approaching policies:

Nurse Advocacy: Adopting a Health in All Policies Approach

Policy advocacy and committed resources are essential to address social factors that shape population health.

https://ojin.nursingworld.org/MainMenuCategories/ANAMarketplace/ANAPeriodicals/OJIN/TableofContents/Vol-23-2018/No3-Sept-2018/Policy-Advocacy.html

Summary

In summary, the diverse field of population health encompasses a range of interconnected components and approaches. It emphasizes the importance of understanding and addressing the health of entire populations, rather than just individuals. Key elements of this framework include primary care, public health surveillance, and public health policy. Community-based participatory research plays a crucial role in population health, involving community members in the research process to better understand local health needs and develop tailored interventions. A culture of health promotes health as a collective goal, fostering a supportive environment for children's and families' wellbeing within communities. Functional medicine in pediatrics emphasizes a holistic approach to children's health, considering both physical, mental, and psychosocial wellbeing. Community-based health education engages communities in health promotion efforts, empowering individuals with knowledge and skills to make healthier choices. Fostering healthy communities is a central goal of population health, with a focus on creating environments that support healthy living. Pediatric population vulnerability recognizes that some children may face unique health challenges due to socioeconomic factors or other social determinants of health. The social determinants of health, such as income, education, and access to healthcare, are critical in understanding and addressing population health disparities. By recognizing and addressing these determinants, population health seeks to improve overall wellbeing and reduce health inequalities on a broader scale. After reading Section 1, learners have a better understanding of how population health is a strong framework for a wellness approach as it relates to the care of children and assists in the transition to Section 2 that discusses population health as it relates children's growth and development.

Credits

IMG 1.1: Copyright © 2012 Depositphotos/pressmaster.

IMG 1.2: Copyright © 2019 Depositphotos/HayDmitriy.

IMG 1.3: Copyright © 2013 Depositphotos/SimpleFoto.

Fig. 1.1: Adapted from Strategies for Quality Care, https://www.strategiesforqualitycare.com/quadruple-aim. Copyright © 2022 by Boehringer Ingelheim Pharmaceuticals, Inc.

Fig. 1.2: Adapted from Brian Castrucci and John Auerbach, "Health Affairs: Meeting Individual Social Needs Falls Short of Addressing Social Determinants of Health," https://debeaumont.org/news/2019/meeting-individual-social-needs-falls-short-of-addressing-social-determinants-of-health/. Copyright © 2019 by de Beaumont Foundation.

Fig. 1.3a: Robert Wood Johnson Foundation, Moving Forward Together, p. 10. Copyright © 2018 by Robert Wood Johnson Foundation. Reprinted with permission.

Fig. 1.3b: Robert Wood Johnson Foundation, Moving Forward Together, p. 4. Copyright © 2018 by Robert Wood Johnson Foundation. Reprinted with permission.

Fig. 1.4: Copyright © 2018 Depositphotos/edesignua.

Fig. 1.5: Leah T. Stiemsma and Karin B. Michels, "The Role of the Microbiome in the Developmental Origins of Health and Disease," *Pediatrics*, vol. 141, no. 4, p. 2. Copyright © 2018 by American Academy of Pediatrics.

Fig. 1.6: Adapted from Build Healthy Places Network, "Fostering Healthy Neighborhoods," https://www.buildhealthyplaces.org/content/uploads/2020/04/Fostering-Healthy-Neighborhoods-Final.pdf, p. 3. Copyright © 2020 by Build Healthy Places Network.

Fig. 1.7: Adapted from National Association of School Nurses, "Framework for 21st Century School Nursing Practice: National Association of School Nurses," *NASN School Nurse*, vol. 31, no. 1. Copyright © 2016 by National Association of School Nurses (NASN).

Fig. 1.8: Source: https://health.gov/healthypeople/priority-areas/social-determinants-health.

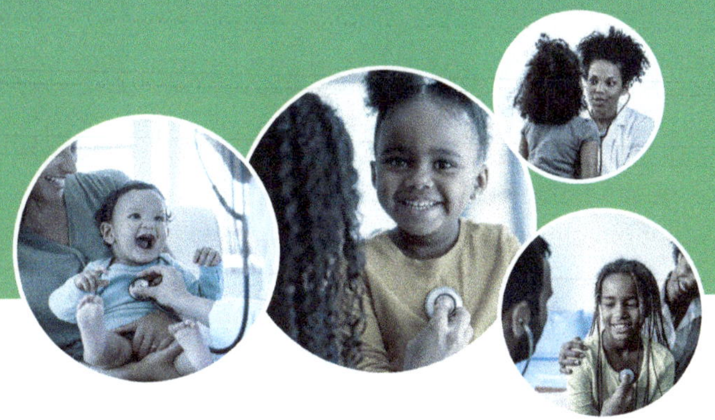

SECTION 2

Growth and Development

Dr. Susan Ward and Frankie Ward, Editorial Assistant

Introduction

From a pediatric population health perspective, understanding the complex connections between wellness and children's health status is essential for promoting optimal growth and development during this critical phase of life. Childhood growth and development are multifaceted processes that encompass physical, mental and psychosocial dimensions. These processes are influenced by a myriad of factors, including, environment, nutrition, healthcare, and socio-economic circumstances. Developmental theories provide a conceptual framework for understanding the growth and developmental processes children undergo. Section 2 will make relevant connections to population health as a framework for understanding children's growth and development. Growth and development across children's lifespan is presented along with a variety of aspects such as vital signs, reflexes, nutrition, temperament, and safety that impact children. Developmental screening and standard developmental theories are also examined. The information presented in Section 2 sets the stage for learners to understand the intricacies

OBJECTIVES

- Discover population health as a framework for understanding growth and development in children.
- Examine the wellness approach as it relates to children's health status.
- Examine growth and development in children across the lifespan.
- Understand vital signs, reflexes, nutrition, temperament, and safety as applied to the care of children.
- Discuss developmental screening used in early identification of children at risk.
- Explore standard developmental theories when comprehending childhood outcomes.

of a population health framework, levels of prevention, health promotion, and legislation and law that directly impact population health found in Section 3.

Population Health Framework

A population health framework plays a pivotal role in fostering growth and development in children. This approach to healthcare and wellbeing prioritizes the collective health of a population rather than solely focusing on individual health outcomes. To support growth and development, a population health framework defines health priorities, offers holistic measures that positively affect health, takes effective measures to eliminate inequities, and improves children's health outcomes. Of course all children are also considered individually, based on their developmental status, to help ensure suitable health outcomes.

Wellness and Children's Health Status

Wellness in children refers to the state of overall health status, wellbeing, and optimal development. A wellness attitude is a multifaceted process that includes creating a way for children to be actively involved in their health patterns (Travis, 1977). Wellness in children and health status are interconnected concepts that focus on the overall health and wellbeing of a community. Both wellness and children's health status adopt a holistic approach to health, considering not only the absence of disease but also physical, mental, social, and emotional wellbeing. In the case of children, this includes growth and development, nutrition, mental health, and access to education and support. Preventive measures and interventions are commonalities in a wellness mindset aimed at improving the health of the entire population. In the context of children, this means promoting healthy behaviors, vaccination programs, regular check-ups, and early intervention to address potential health issues before they become serious. Wellness and children's health status recognize the importance of social determinants of health in shaping outcomes. These determinants include socioeconomic status, access to healthcare, education, safe environments, and supportive communities. Ensuring that children have access to these determinants positively influences their wellness. Both of these concepts also take a long-term perspective, seeking to improve health outcomes over time for the entire population. When applied to children, this means investing in their wellbeing from birth through adolescence, recognizing that early experiences and interventions can have a lasting impact on their health and quality of life. As noted, these ideas are similar to the main premise of a population health framework.

The idea of wellness stems from the 1970s and is still prevalent today. The original wellness continuum is made up of physical, mental, emotional, and social factors that influence health status (Travis, 1977).

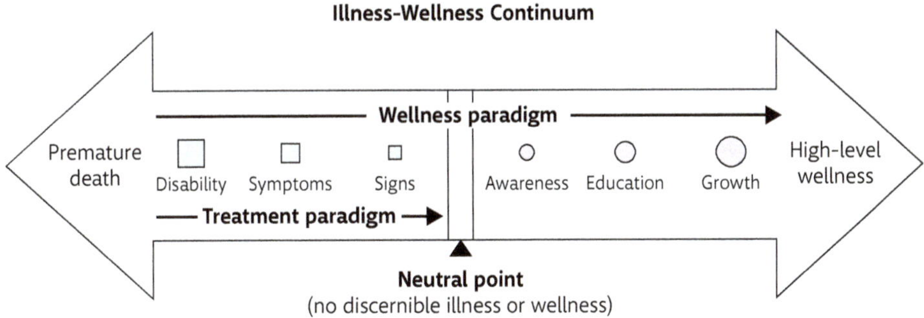

Figure 2.1 Illness–Wellness Continuum

Travis's (1977) illness–wellness continuum proposes individuals move from the left side of the arrow to the right side of the arrow, towards greater health and wellbeing, passing through the stages of awareness, education, and growth. Worsening states of health are reflected by signs, symptoms, and disability (Travis, 1977). Wellness and children's health status extend to their educational experience.

The CDC's (2018c) integrative whole school, whole community, whole child (WSCC) model promotes an association between children's health and education. Collaborative key stakeholders from the fields of health, public health, education, and school health created the model to bring together an approach designed to improve children's learning and health. Established partnerships, including family and the broader community, help secure the necessary resources and the support that children need for holistic development. The WSCC model has 10 main components (CDC, 2018c):

- physical education and physical activity
- nutrition environment and services
- health education
- social and emotional climate
- physical environment
- health services
- counseling, psychological, and social services
- employee wellness
- community involvement
- family engagement

The following textbox includes a link to a website that provides information on the Whole School Whole Community, the Whole Child model (WSCC) that focuses aligning the common goals of public health and school health sectors putting into action an entire approach for children's education.

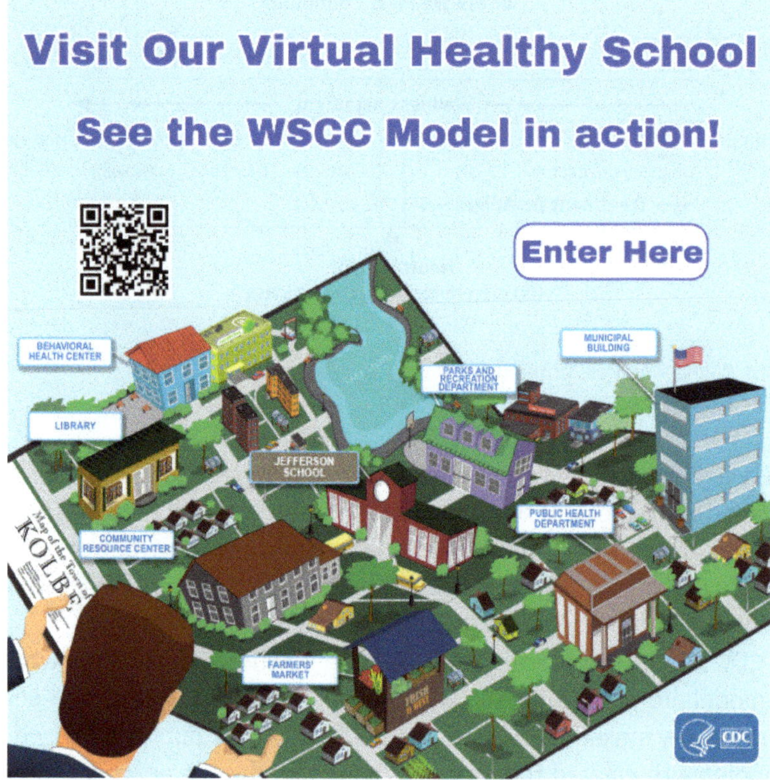

Figure 2.2 The Whole School, Whole Community, Whole Child Model

The Whole School, Whole Community, Whole Child Model

The education, public health, and school health sectors have each called for greater alignment that includes, integration and collaboration between education leaders and health sectors to improve children's development.

https://www.cdc.gov/healthyschools/wscc/index.htm

Growth and Development

Understanding expected growth and developmental aspects in children is essential to the application a pediatric population health framework. Each child grows and develops at their own pace, sometimes moving quickly and at times moving more slowly though the expected stages of development. **Growth** is the constant adjustment in the physical size (internally and externally) of children, while **development** (mental, emotional, social, intellectual, academic, and spiritual) is an ongoing process of adapting to various conditions throughout the lifespan (Ward & Hisley, 2016). Both growth and development are integrated processes, occurring from birth to death. Main considerations of growth and development are cephalocaudal (growth from head to toe), proximodistal (growth from near to far), and gross motor (large muscle groups in the body to perform activities and tasks) and fine motor skills (a category of motor skills that involve the coordination and control of small muscles). For appropriate primary care, it is important to have extensive knowledge of normal expectations for each age group. Growth and development are commonly divided into the following age groups:

- newborn: birth (0 months) to the first month of age
- infancy: 1 month of age to 24 months of age
- toddler: 24 months of age to 36 months of age
- preschooler: 36 months of age to 5 years old
- school-age: 6 years old to 12 years old
- Adolescent: 13 years old to 18 years old

Box 2.1 Developmental Milestones

Developmental milestones are behaviors or skills that illustrate a child's growth in several areas. These milestones are a set of functional skills or age-specific tasks that most children can do at a certain age range. Healthcare providers use milestones to assess how children are developing. Although each milestone has an expected age level, the actual age when a normally developing child reaches that milestone can vary. Every child is unique. The following textbox includes a link to CDC's Developmental Milestones and links to other resources.

CDC's Developmental Milestones

Do you want to download the CDC's free milestone tracker app?

https://www.cdc.gov/ncbddd/actearly/milestones/index.html

Ages and Stages Presented in English and Spanish

The AAP (n.d.-a) website gives growth and developmental information for children from all age groups.

https://www.healthychildren.org/English/ages-stages/Pages/default.aspx

Children of all age groups experience significant growth and development milestones as they journey from infancy to adolescence. During the newborn stage, birth (0 months) to the first month of age, babies enjoy touch as the first sense to develop, have head lag when pulled from a lying to a sitting positon, and randomly grasp caregiver's fingers and objects. In the infant stage, 1 month of age to 24 months of age, infants have an expansive range of growth and development due to the fact that all senses are in tack and well developed. Infants can sit in a tripod position with support, move from crawling, to creeping and eventual walking, and advance from breast or formula feeding to using the pincer grasp; beginning to feed self-finger foods. Toddlers range in age from 24 months of age to 36 months of age and recognize familiar objects, begin running and can hold a large pencil or crayon to make simple marks. Preschoolers are 36 months of age to 5 years old and develop preferences based on use of senses, skip and can hop on one foot and can build a tower of 9–10 blocks. School-age children span from 6 years old to 12 years old and base preferences on the use of senses and improving logic. This age group has better strength, coordination, balance, rhythm, and dexterity and hand-eye coordination. Adolescences span from 13 years old to 18 years old and this period marks the beginning of puberty. Preferences are based on use of senses, improved logic and manipulation of complicated objects. Each age group has its unique challenges and opportunities, but throughout this journey, providing a nurturing and supportive environment is crucial to ensuring healthy growth and development in all aspects of children's lives. Navigate to common questions and concerns that arise during the first months of life textbox for more information.

Common Questions and Concerns that Arise During the First Months of Life

Newborn growth/development information for children 3 months of age is found on the AAP (n.d.-b) website. How a 3 month children should be developing and articles about this age group are included.

https://www.healthychildren.org/English/ages-stages/baby/Pages/default.aspx

Influencing Factors

Influencing factors that may affect the pace and progression of growth and development are based on nature (biological/genetic traits inherent at birth) or nurture (external events such as the environment, health, food, parenting, nutrition, stressors, or schooling). Examples of more significant influencing developmental factors are culture, values, traditions, family patterns, race, ethnicity, or spiritual beliefs. Promoting an environment based on cultural sensitivity is an essential role of the nurse. Remember, growth and development evolve overtime and are holistic—made up of progress in the mind, body, and spirit. Using a pediatric wellness approach and fostering growth and development is paramount in providing safe, competent, and compassionate nursing care. Additional terminology associated with growth and development are growth spurts and anticipatory guidance.

Growth spurts create surges in growth in height and weight. They are a normal part of children's development and occur at different stages during childhood, until they reach physical maturity. Primary care for children includes plotting growth and development over time, achievement of developmental milestones, and understanding that the growth and developmental principles individually apply to each child.

Anticipatory Guidance

Anticipatory guidance is preemptive advice that addresses physical, emotional, psychological, and developmental changes for each age group. Providing information before the next stage of development assists caregivers in understanding the expected growth and developmental parameters. Anticipatory guidance is specific to the aforementioned age groups and its application to population health includes providing information to caregivers to prevent injury, promote disease prevention, and stress benefits of a healthy lifestyle. Common examples of anticipatory guidance per age group include:

- newborn: progress in meeting developmental milestones, frequent healthcare visits, immunizations, sleep patterns, safe environment, communication through crying, nutrition, and bonding
- infant: continued progress in meeting developmental milestones, caregiver response to cries, recognition of early speech patterns ("baby talk" and imitation), immunizations, nutrition, safe environment, and sense of security
- toddler: continued progress in meeting developmental milestones, constant supervision, active exploration of the environment, brief time-outs, immunizations, nutrition, oral hygiene, safe environment, and increased language development
- preschoolers: continued progress in meeting developmental milestones, verbal, and auditory stimulation (talking to, reading, signing), setting limits, safe environment, nutrition, oral hygiene, and school readiness
- school-age: continued progress in meeting developmental milestones, rapid physical and emotional development, immunizations, nutrition, oral hygiene, safe environment, language development, and social development/peer groups
- adolescent: continued progress in meeting developmental milestones, continued rapid physical and emotional development, peer group influence, open lines of communication, immunizations, safe environment, nutrition, oral hygiene, and social development/peer groups

Anticipatory guidance is a pivotal concept in healthcare that has evolved to address the dynamic and complex needs of children across the lifespan. Rooted in preventive care, this proactive approach involves healthcare professionals providing children and caregivers with tailored information and advice regarding potential health risks, developmental milestones, and safety considerations. By anticipating future needs and challenges, healthcare providers can empower children and families to make informed decisions, promote health and wellbeing, and mitigate potential health issues.

The principles, benefits, and applications of anticipatory guidance in healthcare are explored by navigating to the Pediatric Environmental Tool Kit in the textbox.

Anticipatory Guidance

What is anticipatory guidance? Anticipatory guidance assists parents and caregivers in understanding the expected growth and developmental milestones of children. It is commonly seen as learning about the next stage (anticipatory) of development. For instance parents and caregivers learn about toddler milestones when children are nearing the end of infancy.

https://www.atsdr.cdc.gov/emes/training/page19.html#:~:text=Anticipatory%20guidance%2C%20specific%20to%20the,helmets%20and%20to%20use%20sunscreen

A Preventive Approach

Growth and development include a preventive approach of pediatric healthcare as proactive measures that prioritizes the wellbeing of children by identifying potential health risks and intervening early to ensure they thrive. Key principles of preventive pediatric healthcare include:

Early Intervention: Timely identification of health and developmental issues is crucial. Regular well-child visits, starting from infancy, allow healthcare providers to monitor growth, development, and immunization schedules. Early intervention can significantly improve outcomes for conditions such as developmental delays or speech disorders.

Vaccination: Immunizations are among the most effective preventive measures in pediatric healthcare. Following recommended vaccination schedules helps protect children from serious, preventable diseases. Healthcare providers must educate parents and caregivers about the importance of vaccinations and address any concerns they may have.

Health Education: Equipping parents and caregivers with knowledge about child vital signs, reflexes, temperament, and safety are essential topics. Providing evidence-based information empowers families to make informed choices that contribute to a child's overall health and wellbeing.

Nutrition: Regular assessments of a child's growth and nutritional status are fundamental. Identifying and addressing issues such as malnutrition or obesity early can prevent long-term health problems.

Safety: Promoting safety in the home, during play, and while traveling is critical. Healthcare providers should counsel parents on childproofing, car seat safety, and other precautions to reduce the risk of accidents and injuries.

Health professionals in the primary pediatric care setting have a periodicity table of recommendations for preventive pediatric healthcare to guide healthcare practice. This periodicity table identifies routine screenings that should be conducted from the prenatal and newborn stages in infancy through adolescence and into young adulthood at 21 years of age. The categories of the recommendations and timeline include age, history, measurement (e.g., height and weight, head circumference, body mass index, blood pressure); hearing, oral, and vision screenings; developmental social/emotional and behavioral health screenings; substance use, depression, and suicide risk screening; guidance on various laboratory examinations, including hemoglobin, lead, lipid screening, and tuberculosis; and immunizations. Additionally, the social determinants of health compound one another and increase risk of vulnerable pediatric populations, further confirming the need for screenings.

The following link brings the reader to the American Academy of Pediatrics' *Recommendations for Preventative Pediatric Healthcare.* The information stresses children and families are unique; therefore, these the recommendations are designed for children who are receiving nurturing parenting, have no manifestations of any important health problems, and are growing and developing in a satisfactory fashion.

Recommendations for Preventative Pediatric Health Care

These recommendations represent a consensus by the American Academy of Pediatrics (AAP) and Bright Futures.

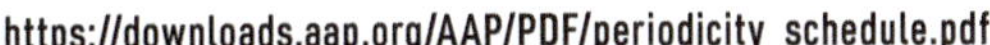

https://downloads.aap.org/AAP/PDF/periodicity_schedule.pdf

Immunizations

The United States has a schedule for childhood vaccines. These vaccines prevent debilitating or life-threatening disease in childhood and beyond. The recommendations followed by the American Academy of Pediatrics are set forth by the Centers for Disease Control and Prevention (CDC). The American Academy of Pediatrics (AAP; 2022) strongly recommends that routine immunizations are administered on the below schedule. The following website shows the importance of having routine access to primary care that provides for regular monitoring of vaccinations.

Recommended Child and Adolescent Immunization Schedule for Ages 18 Years or Younger

View the vaccines needed for the child's and adolescent's immunizations.

https://www.cdc.gov/vaccines/schedules/downloads/child/0-18yrs-child-combined-schedule.pdf

Children's circumstances change and vary overtime. Detailed information helps ensure children are current on vaccines for the child and adolescent immunization schedule. Go to the website below for up-to-date information about the immunization schedule.

Child and Adolescent Immunization Schedule by Age

Read the information on the website for using the schedule and the most up-to-date COVID-19 vaccine recommendations and new or updated recommendations for RSV, Influenza, pneumococcal, polio, and Mpox vaccines.

https://www.cdc.gov/vaccines/schedules/hcp/imz/child-adolescent.html

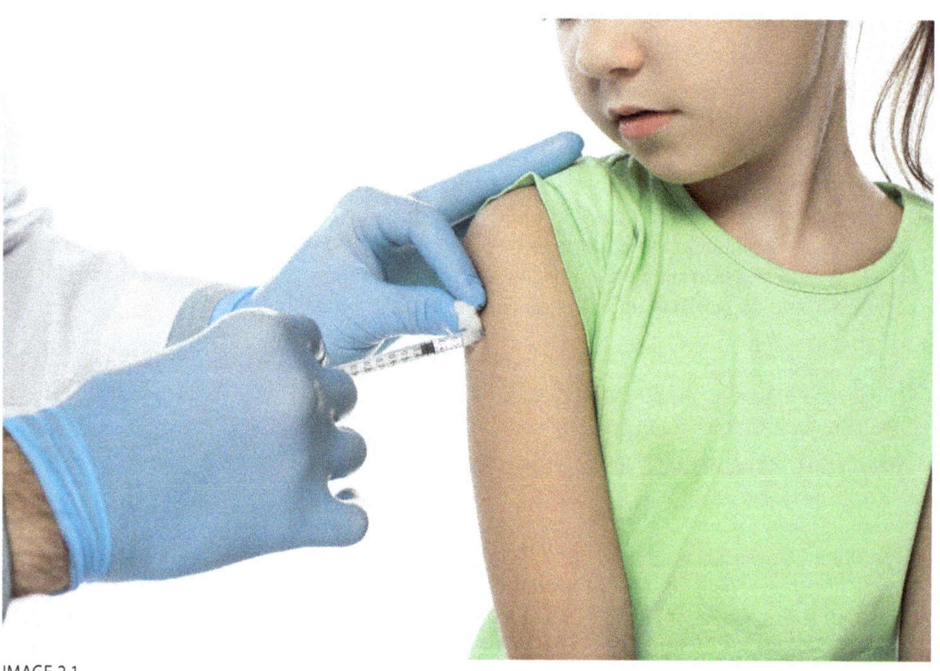

IMAGE 2.1

TABLE 2.1 Children's Growth and Development

Human growth and development are intricate and multifaceted processes that encompass various domains, each contributing to children's overall maturation and wellbeing. These domains collectively shape children's physical growth and sensory development, gross motor skills, fine motor skills, psychosocial development, play, and communication. Navigate to the websites in each age-group to gain more information about growth charts on infants 0 to 2 years and children ages 2 years and older.

GROWTH AND DEVELOPMENT	PHYSICAL GROWTH	SENSORY DEVELOPMENT	GROSS MOTOR SKILLS	FINE MOTOR SKILLS	PSYCHOSOCIAL AND PLAY	COMMUNICATION
Newborn: birth 0 months to the first month of age IMAGE 2.2	Average weight is 7.5 pounds Average height is 21 inches Average head circumference is 13–14 inches Average chest circumference is 12–13 inches **Growth Charts** CDC growth charts ages 0–2 in the United States: **https://www.cdc.gov/growthcharts/index.htm**	Normal newborn sensory days 2–3; baby wakes, cries, and feeds frequently Limited visual acuity (20/100); vision is binocular (sees out of both eyes) Sees bright and contrasting colors Touch is the first sense to develop; newborns love to be touched and cuddled Taste and smell develop in utero, and newborns instantly recognize their mother's smell and breast milk scent (sweet smell) Hearing is developed at birth, and newborns have accurate recognition of familiar voices *See reflexes below Reflexes are present at birth and disappear by 9 months	Absence of head control Head lag when pulled from a lying to sitting a position Body poised in a flexed position (mimics in utero) Rounded back when being held in a sitting position Random movement that is involuntary and erratic Large muscle groups used (kicks legs and waves arms)	Hands are predominantly closed Randomly grasps caregiver's fingers and objects Brings hand(s) to mouth	Normal newborn behavior Day 1, after birth, is alertness for about 2 hours, then baby sleeps to recover from birth Responds to things that give pleasure or discomfort Becoming aware of others Begins to experience separation Fascinated with symmetrical objects (human face) Develops a sense that caretakers are reliable or unreliable Likes to play though touch	Displays emotions through cries Begins to coo/gurgle Smiles involuntarily

(Continued)

GROWTH AND DEVELOPMENT	PHYSICAL GROWTH	SENSORY DEVELOPMENT	GROSS MOTOR SKILLS	FINE MOTOR SKILLS	PSYCHOSOCIAL AND PLAY	COMMUNICATION
Infant: 1–2 months IMAGE 2.3	Weight increases 15 pounds Height increases 1 inch per month Head circumference increases 0.5 inch per month **Growth Charts** CDC growth charts ages 0–2 in the United States: **https://www.cdc.gov/growthcharts/index.htm**	Follows objects and dangling toys with eyes Searches for sounds with eyes Likes to be touched and cuddled Likes sweet taste of breast milk Acute hearing; turns head toward sound	Improved head control Turns head from side to side Less head lag when pulled from lying to sitting Slightly lifts head when in a prone position Movements becoming more purposeful Continues to use large muscle groups	Hands are in an open position Pulls at blankets and clothing Bats at objects in view	Social smile Easily consoled via touch, voice, or gentle movement Likes interactions through play with caregivers Likes imitative games such as patty cake and peek-a-boo	Coos and gurgles Communicates through cries

(*Continued*)

GROWTH AND DEVELOPMENT	PHYSICAL GROWTH	SENSORY DEVELOPMENT	GROSS MOTOR SKILLS	FINE MOTOR SKILLS	PSYCHOSOCIAL AND PLAY	COMMUNICATION
Infant: 3–9 months IMAGE 2.4	Birth weight doubles by 6 months Height increases by 1 inch per month **Growth Charts** CDC growth charts ages 0–2 in the United States: **https://www.cdc.gov/growthcharts/index.htm**	All senses intact and well developed Increased development of binocular vision Beginning hand-eye coordination Follows objects 180° and looks for dropped objects Sees small objects Likes to be touched and cuddled Begins to experience different food flavors Acute hearing; turns head to locate sounds	Holds head more erect Only has slight head lag when pulled to a sitting position Some head bobbing Raises head to 45°–90° when placed on a flat surface Sits in a tripod position with support Some weight bearing when standing with help Rolls from side to side and to abdomen Puts feet in mouth and plays with toes Inspects hands and clutches them together Begins to creep on hands and knees	Grasps and grips objects Shakes rattle Holds bottle Bangs objects together and on surfaces Begins to put objects in container Pulls blanket over face Brings objects to mouth Transfers objects from hand to hand Likes to look at self in mirror	Interacts with caregivers Distinguishes emotions based on voice tone Continues to like interactive games and begins to like songs	Continues to communicate through crying Coos, laughs, uses "baby talk," and has beginning ability to speak "b" and/or "d" sounds (baba or dada) Responds to name

(Continued)

GROWTH AND DEVELOPMENT	PHYSICAL GROWTH	SENSORY DEVELOPMENT	GROSS MOTOR SKILLS	FINE MOTOR SKILLS	PSYCHOSOCIAL AND PLAY	COMMUNICATION
Infant: 9–24 months IMAGE 2.5	Birth weight triples by 9–12 months Height increases by 1 inch per month Head and chest circumference measure the same at 1 year of age **Growth Charts** CDC growth charts ages 0–2 in the United States: **https://www.cdc.gov/growthcharts/index.htm**	Increasing visual depth perception See things at a distance Distinguishes colors Likes to be touched and cuddled Begins to experience different food flavors Acute hearing developed; moves toward sound	Creeps on hands and knees Pulls self up to a standing position and holds on to furniture Begins to stand alone Moves to a sitting position after standing Changes from a prone to a sitting position Takes first steps	Points to objects Begins to show hand dominance Uses pincer grasp; beginning to feed self finger foods Releases objects from highchair and looks for the object Turns pages in a book and rolls a ball	Calms self Interacts with caregivers Begins so show stranger anxiety Begins to explore objects Continues to like interactive games and songs Waves bye-bye	Says "da da," "ma ma," and "uh-oh" Understands a few simple and familiar words Responds to own name

(Continued)

GROWTH AND DEVELOPMENT	PHYSICAL GROWTH	SENSORY DEVELOPMENT	GROSS MOTOR SKILLS	FINE MOTOR SKILLS	PSYCHOSOCIAL AND PLAY	COMMUNICATION
Toddler: 24–36 months IMAGE 2.6	Weight increases 3–5 pounds per year Height increases 3 inches per year **Growth Charts** CDC growth charts for children aged 2 years and older in the United States: **https://www.cdc.gov/growthcharts/index.htm**	Vision well developed Recognizes familiar objects Distinguishes food preferences based on senses Likes to touch different textures Acute hearing; looks for sound coming from another room	Stands and walks independently Begins running Climbs Scoots around on a small tricycle Walks backwards and stands on tiptoes Creeps upstairs and then learns to walk up and down stairs Stands on one foot momentarily Jumps in place	Holds a large pencil or crayon and can make simple marks Turns pages in a book and knobs Begins to feed self with small utensils Removes shoes and socks Drinks from a cup; throws objects on floor Builds tower of 3–4 blocks and knocks over Begins toilet training	Explores and tests boundaries Has tantrums Increased interest in picture books and likes to listen to stories Begins to learn colors and animal sounds Begins parallel play (side by side) Likes interactive games, such as blowing bubbles, tossing a ball, hide and seek, blowing kisses Pulls or pushes toys while walking	Learns new behaviors though imitation Begins to learn cause and effect Follows simple instructions Says single words; knows about 15–20 words Begins to say simple phrases, such as "want drink," "no no," "I do," "go go"

(*Continued*)

GROWTH AND DEVELOPMENT	PHYSICAL GROWTH	SENSORY DEVELOPMENT	GROSS MOTOR SKILLS	FINE MOTOR SKILLS	PSYCHOSOCIAL AND PLAY	COMMUNICATION
Preschool: 36 months –5 years old IMAGE 2.7	Weight increases 5 pounds per year Height increases 25–30 inches per year **Growth Charts** CDC growth charts for children aged 2 years and older in the United States: **https://www.cdc.gov/growthcharts/index.htm**	Senses well developed Develop preferences based on use of senses Colors, textures and noises enhance sensory development Memory improves through sensory experiences	Kicks, throws, and catches a ball Pedals a small tricycle Skips and can hop on one foot Walks down steps, alternating feet Steadily stands on one foot and balances on one foot with eyes closed Jumps on two feet	Builds a tower of 9–10 blocks Draws a stick figure with 6 parts Colors and cuts paper; begins to print letters Uses utensils independently Mostly independent dressing and toileting	Concrete thinking Learns social rules Increased self-regulation Increased confidence; tries new things Associative play (sharing and playing with others) Likes games with rules, interactive games with friends, and pretending	Uses language to convey ideas, requests, and concepts Speaks in complete sentences Recognizes most letters of alphabet Vocabulary of 1,500–2,000 words; asks "why"

(*Continued*)

GROWTH AND DEVELOPMENT	PHYSICAL GROWTH	SENSORY DEVELOPMENT	GROSS MOTOR SKILLS	FINE MOTOR SKILLS	PSYCHOSOCIAL AND PLAY	COMMUNICATION
School-age: 6 years old –12 years old IMAGE 2.8	Weight increases 4–6 pounds per year Height increases 2 inches per year **Growth Charts** CDC growth charts for children aged 2 years and older in the United States: **https://www.cdc.gov/growthcharts/index.htm**	Mature senses 20/20 visual acuity Preferences based on use of senses and use of logic Color discrimination present Senses allow exploration of the environment Talking about how items smell, taste, or feel helps with increased sensory development	Improves in strength, coordination, balance, rhythm and dexterity Likes to climb, bike, and swing Learns to swim, skate, dance, and tumble Balance improves Performs more difficult movements such as twisting, turning or spinning while standing in one place	Good hand-eye coordination Likes activities that promote dexterity, such as arts and crafts, drawing, building models, playing video games, and learning a musical instrument Holds a pencil with a 3 fingered grasp Handwriting improves Ties shoelaces, get dressed, brushes hair and teeth, and gets ready without any help	Increased logical thinking; aware of own thinking and how decisions were reached Solves problems Wants to know “how things work” Understands that actions have consequences Friends become a priority for social interaction Cooperative play; plays in groups Likes sports, interactive games with peers, video and board games, and puzzles	More sophisticated language Increased comprehension Vocabulary of 8,000–15,000 words Enjoys long conversation on a variety of topics

(Continued)

GROWTH AND DEVELOPMENT	PHYSICAL GROWTH	SENSORY DEVELOPMENT	GROSS MOTOR SKILLS	FINE MOTOR SKILLS	PSYCHOSOCIAL AND PLAY	COMMUNICATION
Adolescent: 13 years old to –18 years old IMAGE 2.9	Marks the beginning of puberty Female weight increases 15–55 pounds per year Female height increases 2–8 inches per year Male weight increases 15–66 pounds per year Male height increases 4–12 inches per year All genders develop secondary sex characteristics **Growth Charts** CDC growth charts for children aged 2 years and older in the United States:  **https://www.cdc.gov/growthcharts/index.htm**	Mature senses Preferences based on use of senses and use of improved logic Senses enhance cognitive skills Explores independence through more sophisticated senses	Begins to develop endurance Increases in coordination Develops skills for areas of interest, such as sports, dance, and hobbies Better balance, agility, muscular strength, and endurance	Precise hand-eye coordination Manipulates complicated objects High-level skill set in playing video games Finger dexterity develops for keyboards, writing, repairing, and building	Develops abstract thinking Solves problems using logic Plans for the future Ability to concentrate increases Aware of body image and changes in body Peers are primary social group Begins to explore romantic relationships Continues cooperative play with peer groups, team sports, school, or community activities Enjoys solitary time	Develops adult language Vocabulary of 50,000 words Improves communication skills, including abstract thinking, thought analysis, and problem-solving abilities

From a population health framework, growth and development tables can be tools used for organizing, analyzing, and communicating data about growth and development in a clear and concise manner. These tables serve other important purposes such as visualizing and comparing data, providing a structured framework for presenting the information, and conveying information in as easy to use format to help healthcare professionals and others set priorities. Overtime, tables can track growth and developmental progress and may become a fundamental component of research, policy formulation, and effective communication in various fields.

Vital Signs

Key aspects such as monitoring vital signs, recognizing reflexes, ensuring proper nutrition, understanding temperament, and safety are crucial areas to address in the care of children. Children's vital signs are crucial indicators of overall health status and wellbeing. Vital signs provide essential information about a children's physiological status and help healthcare professionals assess current health condition. Children's vital signs include temperature, heart rate, respiratory rate, blood pressure, and oxygen saturation. Knowing the ranges of children's vital signs provides critical data about overall health status (health promotion/disease prevention measures).

An axillary temperature (using a digital thermometer) or an infrared skin scanner in the temporal area or forehead are the preferred methods of temperature assessment in children due to ease and accuracy. The tympanic route for children older than 6 months is periodically used, but sometimes children do not like the ear pulled (down/back for children younger than 1 year of age and up/back for children over 1 year of age). Oral temperatures are no longer used in children, and rectal temperatures are rarely used but under certain circumstances may be ordered by a healthcare professional. A pulse oximeter reading is also considered a vital sign in children. The oximeter probe is placed on the child's hand or foot, where 95%–100% is a normal oxygen level in healthy children.

TABLE 2.2 Axillary Temperatures

AGE GROUP	CENTIGRADE (°C)	FAHRENHEIT (°F)
Newborn	36.1°C–37.0°C	97.0°F–98.6°F
Infant	36.5°C–37.4°C	97.5°F–99.3°F
Toddler	34.7°C to 37.3°C	94.5°F to 99.1°F
Preschooler	34.7°C–37.3°C	94.5°F–99.1°F
School-age	34.7°C–37.3°C	94.5°F–99.1°F
Adolescent	34.7°C–37.3°C	94.5°F–99.1°F

In the morning, a children's temperature may be as low as 36.3°C (97.4°F) or as high as 37.6°C (99.6°F) in the late afternoon.

TABLE 2.3 Average Range for Vital Signs

AGE GROUP	HEART RATE IN BPM (BEATS PER MINUTE)	RESPIRATORY RATE (BREATHS PER MINUTE)	SYSTOLIC BLOOD PRESSURE IN MMHG (MILLIMETERS OF MERCURY)	DIASTOLIC BLOOD PRESSURE IN MMHG (MILLIMETERS OF MERCURY)
Newborn	120–160	40–60	60–80	30–45
Infant	80–150	25–55	65–100	45–65
Toddler	70–110	20–30	90–105	55–70
Preschooler	65–110	20–25	90–110	60–75
School-age	60–95	14–22	100–120	60–75
Adolescent	55–85	12–18	110–125	65–85

Adapted from Source: Ward, S., & Hisley, S. (2016). Maternal child nursing care: Optimizing outcomes for mothers, children, and families *(2nd ed.). FA Davis, p. 794.*

Reflexes

Reflexes are adaptive and protect newborns during brain and nervous system development. The newborn's reflexes include (Ward & Hisley, 2016):

- rooting: The rooting reflex helps the baby find the breast or bottle and helps prepare them to suck. When the caregiver touches the corner of a newborn's mouth or the baby touches the mother's skin, nipple, or bottle, they turn their head and open their mouth in the direction of the stroking. The rooting reflex in newborns disappears at about 4 months of age and then becomes a voluntary response rather than a reflex.
- sucking: After birth, the sucking reflex is stimulated when the roof of the baby's mouth is placed on the mother's breast or a bottle is offered. The newborn then moves their tongue to suck the breast or bottle. The sucking reflex disappears at about 4 months of age, and then sucking becomes a voluntary response rather than a reflex.
- Moro or startle: In the first 12 weeks of life, the newborn may be startled or surprised by a sudden noise, movement, or bright light. As a response to the trigger, the baby throws their arms out sideways with the palms facing up and tosses the head backwards. The Moro or startle reflex disappears at about 5–6 months of age.
- grasping: Stroking or touching the palm of a newborn causes the baby to automatically close their hands. When a caregiver places their finger in the baby's palm, the baby grasps it and holds on to it. The grasp reflex disappears at about 5–6 months of age.

- Babinski: Firmly stoking the sole of the newborn's foot will cause the big toe to point upward and the other toes to fan out. The Babinski reflex disappears at about 1 year of age.
- stepping: This reflex is also called the walking or dancing reflex. When the baby is held upright with their feet touching a flat surface, they move the legs as if walking or trying to take steps, despite being too young to actually walk. The stepping reflex disappears at about 2 months of age.
- tonic neck: Also known as a fencing reflex, when the baby is supine, the head turns to the right, the right arm stretches out, and the left arm bends at the elbow, forming a "fencing" position. Tonic neck reflex disappears at about 5–6 months of age.

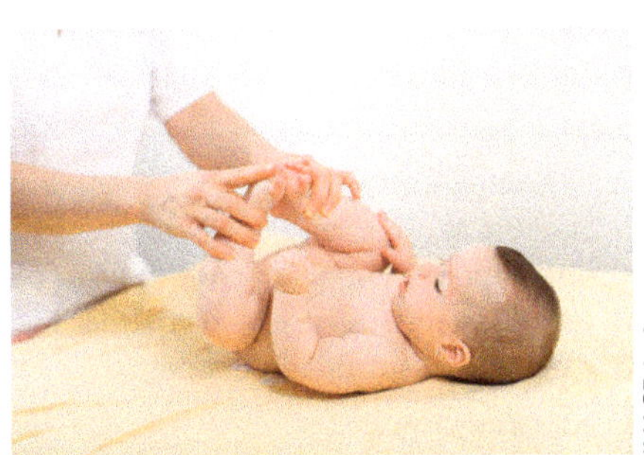

IMAGE 2.10

Nutrition

Following the discussion on reflexes, a conversation about children's nutrition is critically important for several reasons, good nutrition:

- is essential for healthy growth and development
- helps prevent a range of health issues
- impacts the ability to learn and perform well in school
- effects eating habits formed during childhood that persist into adulthood
- helps the body produce antibodies and eliminate pathogens
- provides the necessary energy to maintain an active lifestyle
- promotes overall wellbeing

Nutrition from a population health perspective, informs policy decisions related to food deserts, school meal programs, food labeling, marketing to children, and other initiatives aimed at improving children's access to nutritious food. Socioeconomic factors often play a significant role in determining access to nutritious foods. Ensuring access to proper nutrition for all children is essential for addressing health disparities and promoting health equity. Tailoring nutritional guidance to fit cultural norms and preferences is essential for outcome success.

Good nutrition is particularly important in children's growth and development. Optimal feeding for newborns is breastmilk, and its composition is superior to formula. However, many babies can thrive on formula (Ward & Hisley, 2016). Newborns breast or bottle feed about every 2–3 hours, and as they grow older feeding occurs about every 4–6 hours. At 6–8 months of age, add iron-fortified rice cereal, pureed vegetables, and fruits. By 8–10 months of age, introduce finger foods or mashed foods (including meats). By 1 year of age, allow most table foods, yet still mash or cut them into small bites. Usually, introduce whole milk by 1 year of age (Ward & Hisley, 2016). As children grow, proper nutrition is essential for overall good health. A variety of foods from all food groups—dairy, fruits, cereal and legumes, meat, and vegetables—is recommended. Consider that water is essential, and limit sugary foods. Eating is a complex physical, emotional, and psychosocial experience. A variety of factors play into children's food habits, such as culture, traditions, economic status, health, and preferences (Ward & Hisley, 2016). The following textbox includes a link to USDA My Plate to help children, parents and caregivers learn how to eat healthy.

Learn How to Eat Healthy with MyPlate

Take the My Plate quiz to assess eating habits, find nutrition information on a variety of topics, discover budget friendly food ideas, read about featured items, set personal goals for healthy eating, find easy, low-cost recipes and sign-up for updates.

https://www.myplate.gov/

Temperament

Another key aspect in the care of children is temperament. Responding to and interacting with surroundings, each child displays a unique temperament. Thomas et al. (1968) provide common descriptors that explain children's temperament; regularity (consistency needed), adaptability (willingness to change/adapt to new routines), emotional intensity (strength of reaction to a situation), persistence (willingness to stay engaged in activity regardless of setbacks), distractibility (some difficulty or no difficulty concentrating), mood (disposition), reaction to new people or situations (response, either positive or negative), sensory sensitivity (how senses affect environmental response, low or high), activity level (amount of movement, less or more). Now that some key aspects of child development are covered such as temperament, the information will proceed to discussions on safety and developmental screening.

Safety

Safety is critically important in children's development for several reasons:

- Children's developmental milestones, such as crawling, walking, and exploring, are best achieved in a safe and supervised setting. Safety measures enable children to reach these milestones at an individual pace, which is essential for growth and development.
- Safety measures protect children from physical harm and injuries, which can have long-lasting effects on health and development. A safe environment

reduces the risk of accidents, falls, burns, and other injuries that could impair a child's physical wellbeing.

- Feeling safe and secure is essential for children's emotional wellbeing. A secure and stable environment fosters a sense of trust and helps children develop healthy emotional attachments to parents and caregivers, which is crucial for social and emotional development.
- Safety allows children to explore the environment and engage in age-appropriate activities without fear or anxiety. Feelings of safety promote likeliness to be more curious, ask questions, and engage in learning experiences that promote cognitive development.
- Safety supports positive social interactions. When children are in a safe and nurturing environment, healthy relationships with peers and adults are more apt to develop. A sense of safety can encourage social interaction, cooperation, and the development of essential social skills.
- A safe environment contributes to children's confidence and self-esteem. When children feel secure, a sense of competence and mastery, which is crucial for healthy self-esteem may occur.
- Safety allows children to gradually gain independence and autonomy during interactions with the environment. A secure environment provides the foundation for children to develop self-help skills and a sense of control over personal actions.
- A safe environment reduces stress and anxiety in children. Chronic stress can have detrimental effects on brain development and overall wellbeing. Safety measures help mitigate stressors and create a more relaxed and nurturing environment.
- Safety in childhood can have a lasting impact on an individual's physical and mental health throughout the lifespan. Adverse childhood experiences, including unsafe environments, can lead to negative outcomes in adulthood, such as chronic health conditions and mental health issues.
- Parents and caregivers have a legal and ethical responsibility to ensure the safety of children. Neglecting safety measures can have legal consequences, and it is considered a fundamental aspect of responsible caregiving.
- Safety measures inform public policy via data, evidence, and frameworks that are necessary to advise the development and implementation of public policies aimed at protecting the health, wellbeing, and safety of the public. These measures are essential for addressing risks, preventing harm, and promoting a safer and more secure society. Examples of policies related to safety are disaster preparedness and response, risks and hazards such as lead poisioning that threaten public wellbeing, industry policies for clean air and water, building codes, traffic laws, car seat and helmet saftey and consumer product safety are all informed by public health policies.

In summary, safety is of paramount importance in children's development because it directly influences physical, emotional, cognitive, and social wellbeing. Providing a safe and nurturing environment is a fundamental aspect of caregiving and parenting, as it creates the conditions necessary for children to thrive and reach personal full potential (Safekids Worldwide, 2023).

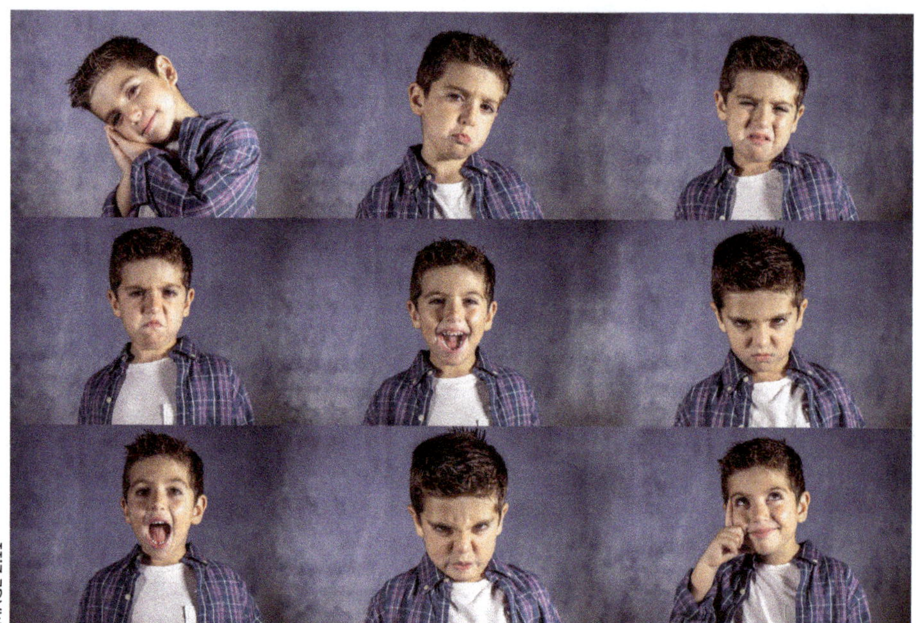

IMAGE 2.11

Developmental Screening

Screening tools provide an effective way to discover evidence of slow or delayed development in young children, up to age 6. **Developmental screening** is used in early identification of children at risk for cognitive, motor, communication, or social-emotional delays. Introduced in 1967, the Denver Developmental Screening Test (DDST) was an excellent source for developmental screening, and an updated version was released in 1992 (DDST II) (Frankenburg & Dodds, 1967; Frankenburg et al., 1992). The screening tool covers four principal areas of development: gross motor, language, fine motor–adaptive, and personal-social.

Screenings may also identify developmental delays that may hinder children's growth, learning, and overall development. Discovered delays may call for further assessment, diagnosis, evaluation, and intervention (Frankenburg & Dodds, 1967; Frankenburg et al., 1992). The following textbox includes a link to Children's Development.

Children's Development Screenings, Milestones, and Suggested Readings
Learn about the Denver II Developmental Screening Test, developmental milestones birth to five years, selected screening and assessment tools and suggested readings on children's developmental norms.

https://www.ccmedical.org/forms/1428352937_171971.pdf

Remember, childhood screening is vital to assessment of expected growth and development. Screening ensures every child a basic premise of population health nursing care. First and foremost, screening serves as an early warning system, allowing healthcare professionals to identify potential developmental delays or growth abnormalities at a stage when interventions can be most effective. Regular screenings, such as those for hearing, vision, and motor skills, enable healthcare providers to track a child's progress and detect any deviations from the expected developmental milestones. This early detection provides parents and caregivers with the opportunity to address any concerns promptly but also ensures that children receive the necessary support and interventions to maximize developmental potential. Go to the textbox below to access the link about the ages and stages questionnaires. Understanding the importance of developmental screenings sets the stage for further knowledge about developmental theories. Another resource in the textbox provides a screening navigator.

Ages and Stages Questionnaires
The website provided information about the ages and stages questionnaires, products and services, an ASQ calculator and screening information.

https://agesandstages.com/

Developmental Theories

Over the course of development, theories explain changes and adaptations children undergo during growth. Developmental theories provide foundational information in understanding childhood outcomes as they relate to population health:

- Parents and caregivers are better equipped to provide appropriate care, support, and guidance to children at each stage of development when informed about developmental theories. For example, knowing about Erik Erikson's stages of psychosocial development can help parents and caregivers navigate issues of trust, autonomy, and identity while fostering a healthier emotional and social development.

- Comprehension of developmental theories may lead to early interventions that allows professionals to recognize developmental delays or deviations from the norm early on. This early identification can lead to timely interventions, therapies, or educational programs that address specific developmental needs, ultimately helping children overcome challenges.
- Awareness of developmental theories is crucial in the field of mental health. It enables mental health professionals to assess and treat children's emotional and behavioral issues with a deep understanding of the underlying developmental factors, leading to more effective and targeted interventions.
- On a larger scale, governments and community organizations can use knowledge of developmental theories to design and implement policies and programs aimed at improving children's outcomes. For instance, programs that address the emotional and social development of at-risk youth may draw from attachment theory or social learning theory to create interventions that are more likely to succeed.

See the textbox for information on developmental theorists and a stages of cognitive development guide.

Child Development Theories and Examples

Understanding developmental theories helps families and community services make more informed decisions regarding the care, education, and support of children. This knowledge contributes to better outcomes by facilitating early intervention, promoting healthy development, and guiding policies and practices that prioritize the wellbeing and potential of children.

https://www.verywellmind.com/child-development-theories-2795068

The source in the previous textbox provides a broad overview of theorists such as Freud, Erikson, Piaget, Bowlby, Bandura, and Vygotsky. Tables 2.4–2.10 and websites offer more information on attachment, psychosocial, cognitive, moral, intelligence, and spiritual theories.

Attachment Theory

Attachment theory, by Mary Ainsworth, is important for several reasons, as it provides valuable insights into human development, relationships, and emotional wellbeing. Attachment theory is a useful way to understand emotional bonds formed by relationships between parents, children and caregivers.

TABLE 2.4 Attachment Theory

DOMAIN	THEORIST/THEORY	IMPORTANT ASPECTS
Attachment	Mary Ainsworth: attachment theory	Infants are born with a need to form a close emotional bond with a caregiver. Attachment is viewed as a progressive bonding process between the mother and infant. The infant's innate temperament and mother's sensitivity towards the child's needs impact attachment (McLeod, 2023a). Attachment becomes instrumental in cognitive, emotional, and social development. **Attachment**  **https://mind.help/topic/attachments/** • A *secure attachment* is described as a bond that is formed when a parent constantly respond to their infant's needs and ensures the child feels secure. The infant is upset when the mother leaves and is happy upon her return (Moretti & Peled, 2004). • *Dismissive-avoidant attachment* occurs when parent's fail to meet the infant's needs. The infant may then see emotional connection as unnecessary. Children manage their own distress and do not signal their need for comfort from the parent. • *Anxious-preoccupied attachment* is associated with inconsistent parenting where the child's bond with their parent tends to be confusing and anxious. The child tends to be difficult to console even when the parent is present. Constant reassurance is needed, yet the child is reluctant to approach the parent for comfort. • *Fearful-avoidant attachment* is considered a disorganized pattern of attachment. Individuals believe they are unworthy of love. It is suspected this attachment is due to severe childhood trauma, emotional neglect, or maltreatment. Children may have extreme and unpredictable behaviors (Ainsworth, 1964; Rees, 2007). The Mind Help (n.d.) website offers more information on attachment (https://mind.help/topic/attachments/).

Maternal Newborn Attachment

Based on the attachment theory provided previously, a specific type of attachment is maternal newborn. Maternal newborn attachment is a priority in the first 1–2 hours after birth and prepares the mother for a positive parenting experience (Holmes et al., 2013; Lauwers & Swisher, 2016). After birth, there are certain stages of newborn adaptation that promotes attachment or bonding (Widstrom et al., 2019):

1. birth cry: The infant lets out an intense cry just after birth, as they are transitioning to breathing air.
2. relaxation: The infant rests activity of mouth, head, arms, legs, or body.
3. awakening: The infant begins to show signs of activity (e.g., small thrusts of head up, down, and from side to side; small movements of limbs and shoulders).
4. active: The infant moves limbs and head in more determined movements. They begin rooting activity, "pushing" with limbs without shifting body.
5. resting: The infant rests, with some activity (e.g., mouth activity, sucks on hand), and this could be interspersed with all the stages.
6. familiarization: The infant has reached areola/nipple with mouth positioned to brush and lick.
7. suckling: The infant has taken nipple in mouth and commences suckling.
8. sleep: The infant closes their eyes and falls asleep.

Sigmund Freud is often regarded as one of the founders of modern psychology. This psychological work laid the foundation for the development of psychotherapy and psychodynamic theories, which have had a lasting impact on the field of psychology.

TABLE 2.5 Freudian Theory

DOMAIN	THEORIST/THEORY	IMPORTANT ASPECTS
Psychosocial	Sigmund Freud: Freudian theory	Influences are biologic instincts and psychosexual in nature.
		Oral stage (1 year of age): The infant's oral curiosity derives pleasure and decreases discomfort by putting objects in their mouth.
		Anal stage (1–3 years of age): The young child learns to control elimination and assert boundaries.
		Phallic stage (3–6 years of age): The child compares male and female bodies, noticing the difference in anatomy. Attraction to the opposite parent is noted (female's fascination of a male caregiver and male's fascination of a female caregivers).

(*Continued*)

DOMAIN	THEORIST/THEORY	IMPORTANT ASPECTS
		Latency stage (6–12 years of age): The older child/adolescent takes a break psychosexually and focuses on growth and learning. *Genital stage* (12–18 years of age): The adolescent experiences the onset of puberty, where the focus is on sexuality, relationships, and a developing sense of romance. Cherry (2022) provides an overview of Sigmund Freud's theories. **Human Behavior** **https://www.verywellmind.com/freudian-theory-2795845**

Psychosocial Development Theory

Erik Erikson's theory extends across the entire lifespan, from infancy to old age, making it relevant to understanding development at all stages of life. This broad and holistic perspective allows for the examination of how individuals navigate and resolve psychosocial challenges at different points in life.

TABLE 2.6 Psychosocial Development Theory

DOMAIN	THEORIST/THEORY	IMPORTANT ASPECTS
Psychosocial	Erik Erikson: stages of psychosocial development	Influences are derived from social interactions. There are eight stages of development that require each stage to be resolved before moving on to the next stage. *Trust versus mistrust* (birth–1 year of age): The infant discovers "Can I trust the people around me?" Trust leads to hope and connection, whereas mistrust leads to hopelessness and disconnectedness. **Psychosocial** **https://www.verywellmind.com/trust-versus-mistrust-2795741**

(Continued)

TABLE 2.6 Psychosocial Development Theory (*Continued*)

DOMAIN	THEORIST/THEORY	IMPORTANT ASPECTS
		Autonomy versus shame and doubt (1–3 years of age): The child discovers "Am I self-sufficient or dependent on others?" Exploration comes with a newfound independence and willpower. Autonomy brings about security and self-confidence, whereas mistrust leads to inadequacy and self-doubt. **Psychosocial**  **https://www.verywellmind.com/autonomy-versus-shame-and-doubt-2795733**
		Initiative versus guilt (3–6 years of age): The child discovers "Am I good or bad?" Initiative brings confidence to try new activities and experiences without excessive fear of failure, which leads to learning to control the environment. If initiative is discouraged, shame ensues and failing to successfully complete tasks occurs. **Psychosocial**  **https://www.verywellmind.com/initiative-versus-guilt-2795737**
		Industry versus inferiority (6–12 years of age): The child discovers "How can I be good?" Industry is developing confidence through proficiency in skills. There is also a sense of pride in accomplishments and abilities. Inferiority leads to lack of confidence and feelings of inadequacy. **Psychosocial**  **https://www.verywellmind.com/industry-versus-inferiority-2795736**

(*Continued*)

DOMAIN	THEORIST/THEORY	IMPORTANT ASPECTS
		Identity versus role confusion (12–18 years of age): The child discovers "Who am I?" The older child/adolescent seeks to establish a sense of self and direction in life. Confusion leads to unsureness about self and may cause a sense of disappointment in life. **Psychosocial**  **https://www.verywellmind.com/identity-versus-confusion-2795735** *Intimacy versus isolation* (19–40 years of age): The young and middle-aged adult discovers "Will I be loved, or will I be alone in life?" Forming fulfilling intimate and loving relationships with others is the focus. Isolation leads to struggling that may result in feelings of loneliness. **Psychosocial**  **https://www.verywellmind.com/intimacy-versus-isolation-2795739** *Generativity versus stagnation* (40–65 years of age): The middle-aged/elder adult discovers "How can I contribute to the world?" Fostering positive changes that may benefit others through societal contributions is important. Stagnant individuals may feel uninvolved, disconnected, or unproductive. **Psychosocial**  **https://www.verywellmind.com/generativity-versus-stagnation-2795734**

(Continued)

TABLE 2.6 Psychosocial Development Theory (*Continued*)

DOMAIN	THEORIST/THEORY	IMPORTANT ASPECTS
		Integrity versus despair (65 years and ends at death): The elder adult discovers "Did I have a meaningful life?" Integrity is a life review that has a sense of accomplishment and fulfillment, whereas despair is described as having feelings of shame, regret, disappointment, or fulfillment. **Psychosocial** **https://www.verywellmind.com/integrity-versus-despair-2795738**

Navigate to the textbox for further information on stages of psychosocial development.

Erik Erikson's Stages of Psychosocial Development

One of the central concepts in Erikson's theory is the notion of identity development. According to Erikson, individuals go through a series of stages, each associated with a specific psychosocial crisis or challenge. Successfully resolving these crises contributes to the development of a strong and cohesive sense of identity.

https://www.simplypsychology.org/Erik-Erikson.html

Jean Piaget's theory of cognitive development is important because it provides a foundational framework for understanding how children learn and grow intellectually. Its influence extends to education, psychology, and child development research, making it a significant contribution to our understanding of human development.

Cognitive Development Theory

Jean Piaget, made significant contributions to the field of developmental psychology with his cognitive development theory. He identified four distinct stages—sensorimotor, preoperational, concrete operational, and formal operational—each characterized by unique cognitive abilities and ways of understanding children's experiences.

TABLE 2.7 Cognitive Development Theory

DOMAIN	THEORIST/THEORY	IMPORTANT ASPECTS
Cognitive	Jean Piaget: cognitive development theory	Main perspectives are based on how children think and learn. There are four distinct phases.

(*Continued*)

DOMAIN	THEORIST/THEORY	IMPORTANT ASPECTS
		Sensorimotor (birth–2 years of age): Primary cognition is experienced through the five senses. Information intake is based on the emotional or physiological factors in the immediate environment. Memory development is recognized through **object permanence**; described as objects and people continue to exist even when they cannot be sensed (seen or heard; Ansorge, 2020). *Preoperational* (2–7 years of age): The focus is mainly on motor skills. There are two substages: preconceptual (thinking about things symbolically) and intuitive (instinctive). There is significant development in the areas of memory and imagination. Increased ability to use actions and words together is evident. Abstract thinking is not yet present. *Concrete operational* (7–11 years of age): Concrete thinking is present. The ability to organize thoughts in a logical order, categorize and label objects, and solve problems is evident. There is more awareness of external events and their impact. The ability to recognize thoughts and feelings becomes important. *Formal operational* (11+ years of age): Uses abstract thinking in problem solving. Ability to analyze two sides of an issue. Thinks systematically and considers multiple possibilities. Ansorge (2020) describes Piaget's stages of development. **Cognitive** https://www.webmd.com/children/piaget-stages-of-development

Moral Development Theory

Lawrence Kohlberg's theory on moral development provides a structured framework for understanding how individuals develop their moral reasoning and ethical decision-making abilities over time. It outlines the stages through which individual's with moral dilemmas, from a focus on self-interest to more abstract principles of justice and ethics.

TABLE 2.8 Moral Development Theory

DOMAIN	THEORIST/THEORY	IMPORTANT ASPECTS
Moral	Lawrence Kohlberg: moral development theory	Focuses on thinking processes involved when making moral decision. Moral development is broken down into three stages. *Level I—preconvention*: The child's moral choices are shaped by the adults' actions and the consequences of following or breaking adults' rules. *Stage 1—obedience and punishment orientation*: The child's behavior is good; thus, they avoid punishment. If the child is bad, they expect discipline because they must have done something wrong. *Stage 2—individualism and exchange*: The child recognizes that there is not just one right point of view. *Level II—conventional*: Conventional morality is characterized by an acceptance of social rules related to right and wrong. Authority is not questioned yet it is internalized. The norms of the group set the standards for reasoning and influence right and wrong views and choices. *Stage 3—good interpersonal relationships*: The child behaves well in order to be seen as a good person. *Stage 4 —maintaining the social order:* The child is mindful of wider societal rules. There is interest in obeying the rules to uphold rules and avoid guilt. *Level III—postconventional*: Individuals understand universal ethical principles. Moral reasoning is based on individual rights and principles of justice. *Stage 5—social contract and individual rights*: The child becomes aware that there are times when rules may work against the interest of others. *Stage 6—universal principles*: Personal moral guidelines are developed that may or may not fit accepted rules. The Simply Psychology website provides information on moral development. **Moral**  **https://www.simplypsychology.org/kohlberg.html#preconventional-morality**

Multiple Theory of Intelligences

Howard Gardner's theory expanded the traditional notion of intelligence, which had been primarily focused on cognitive abilities like logical-mathematical and linguistic intelligence. By identifying multiple forms of intelligence, Gardner acknowledged the diversity of human talents and capabilities, allowing for a more comprehensive understanding of human potential.

TABLE 2.9 Multiple Theory of Intelligences

DOMAIN	THEORIST/THEORY	IMPORTANT ASPECTS
Intelligence	Howard Gardner: multiple theory of intelligences	Individuals have many kinds of intelligences. Several factors influence intelligences, such as cognitive abilities, psychosocial influences, environmental elements, and emotional aspects. There are eight kinds of intelligences. *Naturalistic intelligence* includes individuals who are interested in nature. *Intrapersonal intelligence* includes individuals who are strong in intrapersonal attributes, such as awareness in their own feelings, emotional states, and motivations. *Interpersonal intelligence* includes individuals who are proficient at understanding and interacting with others. *Musical intelligence* includes individuals who have strong musical appreciation and abilities, such as thinking in patterns, rhythms, and sounds. *Bodily-kinesthetic intelligence* includes individuals who have a good perception of body movement, performing, and physical control with good dexterity and hand-eye coordination. *Logical-mathematical intelligence* includes individuals who are proficient at recognizing patterns, reasoning, and logically analyzing problems. Thinking about numbers, relationships, and patterns is a strength. *Linguistic-verbal intelligence* includes individuals who can proficiently use words, both when writing and speaking. These individuals are typically good at writing stories, memorizing information, and reading.

(*Continued*)

TABLE 2.9 Multiple Theory of Intelligences (*Continued*)

DOMAIN	THEORIST/THEORY	IMPORTANT ASPECTS
		Visual-spatial intelligence includes individuals who are proficient at visualization and good with directions, maps, charts, videos, and pictures. The Verywell Mind website provides information on multiple theory of intelligences. **Intelligence** **https://www.verywellmind.com/howard-gardner-biography-2795511**

Stages of Faith

James Fowler's theory provides a comprehensive framework for understanding how individuals develop faith and spirituality over the course of development. It helps explain the psychological and cognitive aspects of faith formation.

TABLE 2.10 Stages of Faith

DOMAIN	THEORIST/THEORY	IMPORTANT ASPECTS
Spiritual	James Fowler: stages of faith	The focus is on changing perspectives of faith through the developmental process. In this model, there are seven primary stages of faith. It is patterned after Erik Erikson's stages of psychosocial development and is in alignment with Jean Piaget's theory of cognitive development. *Stage 0—primal undifferentiated faith* (Birth to 2 years of age): Children's positive experiences with the environment instill feelings of trust and a sense that their surroundings are stable. This sense of security then translates into feelings of trust in the universe and harmony with the divine. In opposition, experiences of maltreatment or neglect may result in feelings of mistrust and fear with the universe and the divine. *Stage 1—intuitive-projective faith* (3–7 years of age): Children's faith is experiential and is developed through the influence of others, stories, images, a sense of what is right and wrong, and their perceptions of how the divine affects the universe. *Stage 2—mythic-literal faith* (7–12 years of age): Children in this stage believe in fairness, justice, and a sense of good and bad. Their image of the divine is someone with human characteristics. Religious symbols and images may be taken literally, which then may cause confusion, leading to a feeling of disappointment with the divine.

(*Continued*)

DOMAIN	THEORIST/THEORY	IMPORTANT ASPECTS
		Stage 3—synthetic-conventional faith (12 years of age to adult): In this stage, the adolescent/young adult has a religious understanding and experiences growth in personal and spiritual identity. When this belief system is challenged, there is a threat to their faith-based identity. *Stage 4—individuate-reflective faith* (mid-20s to late 30s): This stage is sometimes characterized by personal struggle as religious or spiritual beliefs take on greater complexity. The individual may realize potential conflicts between their own belief system and other ways of believing. *Stage 5—conjunctive faith* (midlife crisis): An individual in this stage understands conventional religious traditions yet is also able to grasp a multidimensional perspective, understanding truth cannot be expressed through any one statement of faith. *Stage 6—universalizing faith/enlightenment* (later adulthood): An individual at this stage is not bound by differences in religious or spiritual beliefs but views all people as worthy of compassion and understanding. The American Institute for Learning and Human Development provides information on stages of faith. **Spiritual** **https://www.institute4learning.com/2020/06/12/the-stages-of-faith-according-to-james-w-fowler/**

Developmental theories provide a structured framework for understanding how children change and grow over the lifespan. These theories help explain the processes and patterns of attachment, human behavior, psychosocial, cognitive, moral, intelligence and spiritual development from infancy through adulthood. Parents and caregivers can benefit from developmental theories by gaining a better understanding of their children's needs, behaviors, and capabilities at different ages. Understanding how children learn and develop helps educators tailor instruction to students' developmental needs and abilities. From a population health perspective, policymakers may use developmental theories to inform decisions related to child welfare, education, healthcare, and social services. These theories can guide the development of policies that promote healthy development and wellbeing. Overall, developmental theories have practical applications in parenting, education, policy-making, and research, and contribute to positive population health outcomes for children.

Summary

In summary, Section 2 revolves around understanding children's holistic health and development, and incorporating various facets to ensure wellbeing. A population health perspective considers the broader physical and psychosocial factors that impact children. The wellness approach and its relevance to children's health emphasizes not merely the absence of illness but also the promotion of overall wellness. Examining growth and development in children across the lifespan includes comprehending the various stages and milestones children go through from infancy to adolescence. Key aspects such as monitoring vital signs, recognizing reflexes, ensuring proper nutrition, understanding temperament, and safety are crucial areas to address in the care of children. Developmental screening for early identification highlights the importance of using screening tools for early identification of children at risk. These screenings help identify potential developmental delays or issues in children, enabling timely intervention and support. The exploration of standard developmental theories give insights into childhood outcomes. By understanding these theories, healthcare professionals can better anticipate and address the developmental needs and challenges children may face.

Overall, the topics Section 2 collectively contribute to a comprehensive approach to child health and development, considering both individual and population-level factors to promote the wellbeing of children through growth to maturity. After reading Section 2, learners have a better understanding about how population health is a strong framework for understanding growth and development in children and assists in the transition to Section 3 that discusses levels of prevention, health promotion with guidance in finding accompanying resources in the context of pediatric care.

Credits

Fig. 2.1: John W. Travis and Regina Sara Ryan, "Illness-Wellness Continuum," *The Wellness Workbook: How to Achieve Enduring Health and Vitality*, Celestial Arts Publishing Company, p. xviii. Copyright © 2004 by John W. Travis.

Fig. 2.2: Source: https://www.cdc.gov/healthyschools/wscc/index.htm.

IMG 2.1: Copyright © 2020 Depositphotos/IgorVetushko.

IMG 2.2: Copyright © 2014 Depositphotos/halfpoint.

IMG 2.3: Copyright © 2022 Depositphotos/PeopleImages.com.

IMG 2.4: Copyright © 2022 Depositphotos/spongePo.

IMG 2.5: Copyright © 2012 Depositphotos/Gelpi.

IMG 2.6: Copyright © 2010 Depositphotos/erierika.

IMG 2.7: Copyright © 2019 Depositphotos/ramirezom.

IMG 2.8: Copyright © 2015 Depositphotos/Wavebreakmedia.

IMG 2.9: Copyright © 2017 Depositphotos/TarasMalyarevich.

IMG 2.10: Copyright © 2012 Depositphotos/Lighthunter.

IMG 2.11: Copyright © 2019 Depositphotos/coscaron.

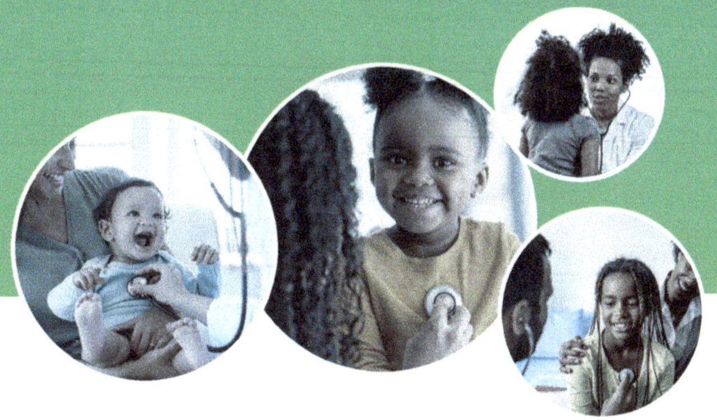

SECTION 3

Levels of Prevention and Health Promotion

Dr. Alice Kindschuh, Dr. Kiley Petersmith, Dr. Susan Ward, and Frankie Ward, Editorial Assistant

Introduction

In today's rapidly evolving healthcare landscape, a holistic approach to children's wellbeing is paramount. It involves not only addressing children's immediate medical needs but also delves into the broader context of population health and the multifaceted challenges children may face. In section 3, a deeper dive into exploring the intricacies of a population health framework, levels of prevention and health promotion with guidance in finding accompanying resources and mental health in the context of pediatric care is presented. Additionally, legislation and law that play a crucial role in shaping policies and regulations that directly impact population health are offered. The elements in this section collectively contribute to a comprehensive and compassionate approach to safeguarding the wellbeing of children, who represent the future and the heart of any society. Section 3 prepares learners for Section 4, found on Cognella Active Learning that has interactive exercises, case studies, critical thinking exercises, Next Generation NCLEX style questions, and math questions.

OBJECTIVES

- Discover population health as a framework for children related to the health of the community.
- Investigate health promotion for improvement in the overall health outcomes of children.
- Understand the main intention of prevention.
- Explore a detailed approach to primary, secondary, and tertiary levels of prevention.
- Comprehend mental health strategies related to primary prevention.
- Critique legislation and law as a legal framework for regulating public health practices.
- Acquire guidance on primary, secondary, and tertiary prevention resources.

Population Health Framework

The focus of a population health framework for children is to address health and wellbeing within the context of the broader community. This framework takes into account various factors that can influence children's health outcomes and aims to improve the overall health and quality of life. Some key aspects that a population health framework for children typically focuses on are preventive healthcare, social determinants of health, health equity, early identification and interventions, community-based approaches, a holistic view, family-centered care, cultural sensitivity, health disparities and data and research.

Prevention includes promoting healthy behaviors, immunizations, and early interventions to prevent the onset of health issues in children. Social determinants of health recognizes that children's health is influenced by social determinants such as socioeconomic status, access to education, housing conditions, and community environments. Addressing these social determinants is crucial for improving child health outcomes. Health equity places a strong emphasis on ensuring that all children, regardless of background or circumstances, have equal access to healthcare services and opportunities for better health. Early identification and interventions for health and developmental issues in children are a key focus because timely interventions can prevent health problems from becoming more severe and can improve long-term outcomes.

A population heath framework also emphasizes the importance of community-based approaches to children's health. This involves collaboration among healthcare providers, schools, social services, and community organizations to create a supportive environment for children's health and wellbeing. This framework takes a holistic view of children's health, considering not only physical wellbeing but also mental and psychosocial health. It recognizes that these aspects are interconnected and impact overall health.

Family-centered care and support are integral to the framework. Recognizing that families play a vital role in children's health because it promotes a family-centered care approaches that engage and empower parents and caregivers. Cultural sensitivity is acknowledged, and efforts are made to provide culturally sensitive healthcare and support services that respect the diverse backgrounds and needs of children and families. The population health framework seeks to reduce health disparities among children, particularly among vulnerable or marginalized populations, by addressing the root causes of these disparities and ensuring equitable access to healthcare services.

Finally, data and research are essential components of a population health framework for children. Gathering data on child health trends, risk factors, and outcomes helps in making informed decisions and developing effective interventions. In essence, a population health framework for children focuses on a comprehensive and proactive approach to children's health, with the goal of promoting wellness, preventing illness, and improving the health and wellbeing of all children within a given population. It recognizes that the health of children is interconnected with the health of the community and society as a whole, making it a crucial component of public health efforts (Wilson & Jovanovic et al., 2019; Bhattacharya & Bhatt 2017).

Population Health Framework

The focus of a population health framework is on primary prevention for children who may be at risk to develop physical, mental, or psychosocial conditions. In a population health model, health care professionals can intervene to impact several conditions:

- childhood screenings
- childhood vaccinations
- developmental milestones
- hand hygiene/germ prevention
- childhood obesity
- education about tobacco use
- dental care/fluoride supplementation
- education about safe sex/birth control
- pediatric resource recommendations

Health Promotion

The ultimate aim of health promotion is to reduce the burden of preventable diseases rather than simply treating them once they have developed, improve the overall health of populations, and enhance the quality of life for children, families and communities. Health promotion focuses on providing families and communities with accurate and accessible information about health risks and benefits to help make informed decisions about health. Health promotion efforts can take many forms, including health education campaigns, policy changes, workplace wellness programs, and community-based interventions.

Encouraging families to adopt healthy behaviors and lifestyles, such as eating a balanced diet, and engaging in regular physical activity will promote better health outcomes. Empowering families to take control over their own health by providing them with the necessary skills and resources to make healthy choices will enhance self-care. Families must also recognize that social, economic, and environmental factors have a significant impact on health and addressing these determinants will reduce health inequities. Emphasizing preventive measures, such as vaccinations, regular screenings, and early detection to identify health issues before these conditions become more serious is paramount in health promotion. Involving families in the planning and implementation of activities may ensure activities are culturally appropriate and tailored to individual needs.

Health promotion focuses on population-based initiatives and policies. According to the WHO (2016), health promotion activities enable a population to attain health through a range of social and environmental policies. Health promotion advances health and quality of life by addressing the root causes of illness by empowering individual and population controls to promote healthy behaviors (WHO, n.d.). Promoting policies and advocating for changes at the community, national, and global levels that support and enable healthy choices and environments is essential in the health promotion mind-set. Communities can work with various stakeholders, including healthcare professionals, educators, government agencies, non-profit organizations, and communities, to develop and implement health promotion programs and initiatives. Striving for equitable access to healthcare and health-promoting resources for all individuals, regardless of background or socioeconomic status is key in health promotion. (Office of Disease Prevention and Health Promotion, n.d.-a; Office of Disease Prevention and Health Promotion, n.d.-b; Office of Disease Prevention and Health Promotion, 2022; World Health Organization, n.d).

Health promotion and primary prevention have similar key components and are upstream approaches to population health. Secondary and tertiary, or downstream, prevention occur after illness or disease has occurred. Upstream and downstream approaches are instrumental in population health, but the more resources dedicated to upstream, the fewer resources are needed downstream.

Disease Prevention

It is important to differentiate health promotion and disease prevention, as while the concepts are interrelated, there is a distinct difference. **Disease prevention**, whether it is for an individual or a population, addresses the risk factors associated with disease and minimizes the burden of disease (WHO, n.d.). Disease prevention efforts often occur within healthcare (WHO, n.d.). Disease prevention efforts intervene through education and support before health effects occur (e.g., altering risky behaviors, using tobacco, or eating poorly).

Levels of Prevention

The main intention of prevention is to decrease risk for disease and injury (Institute for Work and Health, 2015). Central to the idea of a prevention is assisting populations in overcoming barriers, connecting to resources, and achieving increased access to services. Prevention occurs through partnerships that develop health promotion education programs. To effectively protect the health of children, it is imperative to examine the three levels of prevention: primary, secondary, and tertiary. Primary prevention seeks to prevent the onset of health issues by addressing risk factors and promoting healthy behaviors. Secondary prevention focuses on early detection and intervention, aiming to minimize the impact of existing conditions. Tertiary prevention is centered on managing and mitigating the effects of chronic conditions, preventing complications, and enhancing the quality of life for affected children. Understanding these levels of prevention is essential to implementing a comprehensive approach to pediatric population health. Navigate to the textbox to read important information about prevention.

> **Picture of America**
> Picture of America provides detailed information about a prevention framework and its key components.
>
> 
>
> **https://www.cdc.gov/pictureofamerica/pdfs/picture_of_america_prevention.pdf**

Primary Prevention

Primary prevention focuses on prevention of the development of disease and illness and the prevention of injury. It typically focus on addressing root causes and risk factors associated with a particular health issue. The strategies promote not only the physical health of children but also social and economic health. Other primary prevention strategies include screening and early detection, health education, immunizations, environmental, safety measures, lifestyle modifications, health promotion programs, and policy and legislation initiatives. For example, a primary prevention strategy is an antipoverty and family support program, especially when combined with health programming, which may have a considerable positive influence on the health of communities. It is also a crucial component of public health, as it can reduce the burden on healthcare systems. (Institute for Work and Health, 2015).

What are the advantages of using primary prevention resources?

- Cost-Effective: Primary prevention is often more cost-effective than treating diseases or addressing issues after the conditions have already developed. It can save healthcare systems, governments, and individuals substantial financial resources by avoiding the high costs associated with medical treatment, rehabilitation, and long-term care.
- Promotes Health and Well-Being: Primary prevention resources focus on promoting overall health and wellbeing by addressing risk factors and promoting healthy behaviors. This approach not only prevents specific diseases or issues but also contributes to a healthier population.
- Enhances Quality of Life: By preventing diseases and social problems, primary prevention resources help children and families lead healthier lives. The burden of illness, disability, and suffering is reduced, leading to improved quality of life for families and communities.
- Reduces Mortality: Many diseases and health conditions can be life-threatening if left untreated or undetected. Primary prevention measures, such as vaccinations, health education, and lifestyle interventions, can significantly reduce mortality rates by preventing these conditions from occurring in the first place.

- Promotes Equity: Primary prevention resources can be designed to target vulnerable populations, such as children and families and address health disparities. By focusing on prevention, these resources aim to reduce the unequal problem of disease and social issues among different demographic groups.
- Long-Term Impact: Primary prevention may have a lasting impact on health and wellbeing. Once children and families adopt healthier behaviors or receive vaccinations, the benefits continue throughout life, reducing the risk of future health problems.
- Prevents the Spread of Diseases: Primary prevention resources are crucial in halting the spread of infectious diseases. Immunization campaigns, for example, prevent epidemics by establishing herd immunity, reducing the number of susceptible individuals in a population.
- Empowers Children and Families: Primary prevention resources empower children and families with knowledge and tools to take control of personal health. Health education and awareness campaigns provide children and families with the information needed to make informed decisions about lifestyle choices.
- Reduces the Burden on Healthcare Systems: Preventing diseases and social issues at the primary level reduces the demand on healthcare systems, allowing the allocation of resources to be used more efficiently and effectively (Institute of Medicine (US) Roundtable on Evidence-Based Medicine, 2010).

Primary Prevention Examples

Following, there are several examples of primary preventions where organizations are working collaboratively for children and families addressing health, housing, poverty, and other social sectors that demonstrate positive outcomes in unique structures and processes. The following textbox includes a link to the Women, Infants, and Children website.

WIC—Women, Infants, and Children

The federal program Special Supplemental Nutrition Program for Women, Infants, and Children (WIC) supports low-income mothers, children, and infants with food and formula.

https://dhhs.ne.gov/Pages/WIC.aspx

Vaccinations

Childhood immunizations and vaccines are a commonly addressed as a primary prevention measure for several reasons such as to prevent disease before exposure, protect vulnerable populations, give long lasting protection, decrease cost, reduce disease burden, and eradicate devastating diseases (e.g., smallpox). Missed or delayed routine childhood immunizations create the potential for the risk of infectious diseases and other outbreaks of previously preventable and controlled diseases like measles, polio, or pertussis. Identifying opportunities in promotion and continuation of childhood vaccination programs has come to the forefront in population health initiatives. The following resources highlight tools and programs that can facilitate timely vaccination.

Vaccinations

This resource from the CDC is a call to action to add routine and COVID-19 vaccinations to the back-to-school checklist.

https://www.cdc.gov/vaccines/hcp/clinical-resources/downloads/safe-return-school.pdf

The Vaccines for Children (VFC) program provides free vaccines for children. The following resource offers information on eligibility and access to the program.

https://www.cdc.gov/vaccines/programs/vfc/parents/qa-detailed.html

One consequence of COVID-19 was that many children became behind on vaccinations and missed regular check-ups. This resource helps parents get back on track.

https://www.cdc.gov/vaccines/parents/visit/vaccination-during-COVID-19.html

COVID-19 Pandemic

The COVID-19 pandemic highlighted devastating and disproportionate ill health effects of structural racism and unmet social need, while amplifying a message that has since led to policy development and funding that aid in addressing the SDOH. The COVID-19 pandemic overburdened an already existing crisis impacting the complex needs of children related to their physical, social, emotional, and mental wellbeing. Compounding overall health for children is lack of housing, inadequate safety and protection, and poverty. To address pediatric health from a population health lens, healthcare providers must reduce and mitigate significant Adverse Childhood Experiences (ACEs) and do so in the environment where children live, learn, and play (Centers for Disease Control and Prevention, 2021).

Life Course Intervention Visual Toolkit

The Life Course Research Visual Toolkit YouTube channel focuses on when and how to influence an individual's life course and promote positive health outcomes. This toolkit views children and families through a holistic lens, focusing specifically on family health, early childhood mental health, adversity and resilience, and school. This toolkit helps guide health care practitioners to understand how health and disease emerges over the course of a lifespan. In the textbox, click into the website for a variety of resources you can choose from the Life Course Research Visual Toolkit.

The Life Course Research Visual Toolkit

The Life Course Research Visual Toolkit gives examples on the complexity of how disease and health outcomes influence the course of a lifespan. Choose the topics that interest you the most.

https://www.youtube.com/channel/UCoLmkCnGcvGVM8HhYF6hoSg

Eliminating Racism and Empowering Women in the Tri-County Area

Learn more about intersectional programming on the YWCA Tri-County Area website.

https://www.ywcatricountyarea.org/what-we-do/

YWCA

The Pennsylvania YWCA Tri-County Area program focuses on urgent action to develop equity-focused, community-driven programming in preventing and healing adverse childhood trauma and supporting historically marginalized communities. The success of this project has evolved into early educational opportunities, including age-appropriate milestone assessment, behavioral support, as well as providing daily meals/snacks before and after school. This community organization partners with other area entities to aid with rent and utilities. The information includes other programming sessions on youth empowerment strategies, foster grandparents, and advocacy initiatives. Additionally, there is information on education, social justice, racial inequities, and safe healthy communities. The following link brings the reader to the YWCA Tri-County website.

Federally Qualified Health Centers

A key role of federally qualified health centers (FQHCs), health services within community education centers, is to provide programs addressing safety and obesity and strategies that support mental health of children and other vulnerable pediatric populations. Another critical function is to serve the population holistically by providing physical, mental, and social resources in one location. FQHCs purposefully reach out to uninsured or underinsured populations by offering a sliding fee scale and providing comprehensive services, including:

- transportation services necessary for adequate patient care
- preventive health services and well-child services
- mental health and substance abuse services
- hospital and specialty care
- dental services

The following textbox includes a link to Health Resources and Services Administration (HRSA).

HRSA Find a Health Center Tool
Use this tool to find qualified health centers for community referrals.

https://findahealthcenter.hrsa.gov/

School-Based Health Centers

A school-based health center in Rhode Island partnered with the Neighborhood Health Plan of Rhode Island, a nonprofit health maintenance organization, to incentivize and encourage students to enroll in and receive a physical exam within a school-based health center. The partnership and gift incentive resulted in a 40% increase in the number of adolescents 13–16 years of age who received a complete physical exam (Centers for Medicare and Medicaid Services, 2014).

Head Start

Head Start is an example of a community organization categorized in both primary and secondary prevention levels. It is made up of comprehensive community education options that promote school readiness by offering educational, nutritional, health, social, and other services to young children in low-income families. The services are available from birth to 5 years old. A key element of this program is the effort to actively engage parents in services to achieve strong child outcomes by encouraging learning through play, supporting cultural and language heritage of families, creating indoor and outdoor learning environments, and performing ongoing assessments for progress. Child and family health, wellbeing, and engagement are at the core of the programming. Children must have annual health screenings, which includes a physical exam, dental exam, lead and hemoglobin screening, and hearing and vision screening. Programs are also designed to address community needs as indicated through community needs assessments. The following textbox includes a link to the Head Start Center locator.

Early Child Education and Knowledge Center's Head Start Program
Use the following resource to find local Head Start Centers.

https://eclkc.ohs.acf.hhs.gov/center-locator

Nursing College Collaborates with Local Community Agency

Dr. Kiley Petersmith, director of the Center for Diversity and Community Engagement at Nebraska Methodist College (NMC), decided to partner with a local community agency. Specific areas of support include addressing failed or missed well-child visits, financial hardship, transportation barriers, behavioral health, and physical health concerns such as asthma and ear infections. Throughout the clinics, families are screened for SDOH risk factors and children receive developmental milestone surveillance. The screening aims to identify unmet physical and social needs, assess children's growth and development, and provide needed resources. Each year approximately 100 children living in homeless and unhoused situations are evaluated, and referrals of 350–400 distinct health needs for the approximately 100 children are made based on surrounding health, growth and development, housing, safety, and nutrition. Referrals include:

- primary care
- lead and hemoglobin screenings
- routine immunizations
- dental exams
- vision exams
- behavior evaluation
- speech therapy evaluation
- food support
- transportation assistance
- ear, nose, throat referrals for recurrent infections

Navigate to the next website to learn more about this population health initiative.

Population Health Initiative

The outcomes of this project include addressing social and environmental determinants, developing community partnerships, coordinating outreach initiatives of screening, and reducing the barriers of access to healthcare.

https://www.methodistcollege.edu/about/community

Mental Health

Primary prevention in relation to mental health focuses on strategies and interventions aimed at preventing mental health problems and promoting psychological wellbeing before occurrence of mental health issues. Primary prevention focuses on proactively addressing risk factors, promoting protective factors, and fostering resilience to prevent the onset of mental health problems. Some of the important benefits of primary prevention in the context of mental health include: they promote emotional and social development, reduce mental health disorders, increase the ability to cope with life stressors and challenges, improve overall wellbeing, provide a positive impact on academic performance, reduce stigma and contribute to stronger and more resilient communities. See the following American Academy of Pediatrics (AAP), Healthy Children.org website for good resources that provide strategies on how to talk about mental health concerns with children and adolescents.

A prevalent issue among adolescents is anxiety, depression, and other mental health concerns. The AAP joined with other organizations to declare a national emergency in youth mental health. Children, adolescents, and families may need added support in talking about mental health concerns with a healthcare provider. When mental issues occur and impact daily routines, it could be a sign of a more serious mental health concern. Go to the website for information about how to talk about children's mental health concerns.

Teen Mental Health: How to Know When Your Child Needs Help

Use the following resource to learn more about the issue of child and adolescent mental health.

https://healthychildren.org/English/ages-stages/teen/Pages/Mental-Health-and-Teens-Watch-for-Danger-Signs.aspx

Mental Health in the Classroom

Promoting children's mental health in the classroom is essential for overall wellbeing, emotional development, and academic success. There are several tools and strategies that educators and school professionals can use to support children's mental health at school. Additionally, creating a stigma-free and empathetic classroom culture where students feel safe discussing emotions is essential for the success of these efforts. It's important for educators and other health care professionals to be aware of and trained in these tools and strategies to effectively support children's mental health in the classroom:

How to Talk About Mental Health with Your Child and the Pediatrician

Mental health concerns have become an important aspect of well-child visits.

https://healthychildren.org/English/healthy-living/emotional-wellness/Pages/How-to-Talk-with-Your-Child-and-Their-Pediatrician-About-Mental-Health-Concerns.aspx

- Positive Behavior Support (PBS) Programs: PBS programs are designed to create a positive and supportive classroom environment. They emphasize proactive strategies for managing behavior, teaching social skills, and reinforcing positive behaviors rather than focusing solely on punishment.
- School-wide Positive Behavior Interventions and Supports (PBIS): PBIS is a framework that emphasizes positive behavior reinforcement throughout the entire school. It involves setting clear expectations, providing consistent consequences, and recognizing and rewarding positive behavior.
- Social-Emotional Learning (SEL) Curriculum: SEL programs are specifically designed to help children develop essential social and emotional skills, such as self-awareness, self-regulation, empathy, and interpersonal communication. Implementing an SEL curriculum can promote emotional intelligence and improve classroom behavior.
- Early Intervention: Identifying and addressing mental health concerns early is crucial. Schools can have systems in place to recognize signs of distress and refer students to appropriate services or interventions.

- Counseling and Support Services: Schools often have counselors or mental health professionals who can provide individual or group counseling to students. These professionals can help students address emotional and behavioral challenges.
- Parent and Caregiver Involvement: Collaboration with parents and caregivers is crucial. Schools can offer workshops and resources to help families support children's mental health at home.
- Mindfulness and Relaxation Techniques: Teaching children mindfulness and relaxation exercises can help them manage stress and anxiety. Simple practices like deep breathing, guided imagery, or short mindfulness exercises can be integrated into the daily routine.
- Classroom Behavioral Management Strategies: Teachers can implement various strategies to create a positive classroom environment, such as clear and consistent expectations, positive reinforcement, and a calm and structured routine.
- Flexible Seating and Learning Environments: Providing flexible seating arrangements and learning spaces can accommodate different learning styles and sensory needs, contributing to a more comfortable and inclusive classroom environment.
- Emotion Regulation Tools: Providing tools like sensory objects or emotion regulation cards that children can use when needed to calm down or express emotions in a constructive way.
- Peer Support and Peer Mediation: Encouraging peer support and teaching conflict resolution skills can help students build positive relationships and resolve conflicts in a healthy manner.
- Classroom Meetings: Regular classroom meetings where students can discuss feelings, concerns, and ideas can promote a sense of community and give students a platform to voice personal thoughts.
- Educational Technology: Educational apps and software are designed to promote emotional regulation and mental health. These tools may offer exercises, games, or guided activities that help children manage stress and anxiety.
- Trauma-Informed Practices: Schools can adopt trauma-informed approaches that take into account the potential trauma that some students may have experienced. This involves creating a safe and supportive environment and providing appropriate resources for trauma-affected children.
- Monitoring and Evaluation: Regularly assess and monitor the mental health and emotional wellbeing of students through surveys, observations, and discussions with school professionals.

Navigate to the website below for information and tools to be used in the classroom.

Kids' Health in the Classroom

Nemours Tools for Healthy Schools provides a toolkit of resources for classroom K–12 educators to bring age-appropriate preventative health and wellness information and activities to kids while at school.

Healthy Schools

The toolkit is divided by age and is available in multiple languages.

https://classroom.kidshealth.org/classroom/

The Collaboratory for Kids and Community Health

The Nationwide Children's Hospital has created a Collaboratory for Kids and Community Health hub for innovative ideas addressing the health of children in neighborhoods, the inequalities, and mental and behavioral health as well as how to advance health while saving money. Go to the textbox for innovative ideas improving the health of children and neighborhoods.

The Collaboratory for Kids and Community Health

This hub has resources, toolkits, and example programs from around the United States that are working together to create change.

https://www.nationwidechildrens.org/about-us/collaboratory

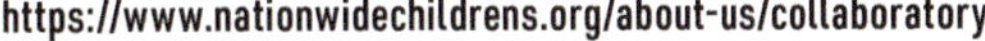

Legislation and Law

Legislation provides a legal framework for regulating public health practices. It is the process of creating, drafting, and the formal act of making or enacting laws. It is carried out by legislative bodies such as parliaments, congresses, or assemblies at the federal, state, or local levels of government. During the legislative process, proposed laws, known as bills, are introduced, debated, amended, and ultimately voted on by the legislative body. Using a population health framework, legislation enables governments to set and enforce standards for various aspects of health, including sanitation, food safety, air and water quality, and workplace safety.

Laws, on the other hand, are the actual rules, regulations, and provisions that govern society. They are the legal rules that individuals and organizations must follow. Laws are the result of successful legislation. When a bill is passed by a legislative body and signed into law by the relevant authority (i.e., the president, governor, or mayor), it becomes a law. Laws often focus on prevention, health equity, and the social determinants of health. Laws can cover a wide range of subjects such as the Affordable Care Act, the Clean Air and Water Act, National Childhood Vaccine Injury Act (NCVIA) and, the Americans with Disabilities Act (ADA). Legislation and law are essential for preventing the spread of diseases and reducing health risks for everyone, including children and families.

Legislation

- Legislation can be used to address health disparities and promote health equity. Laws can require equitable access to healthcare services, funding for underserved communities, and measures to reduce the social determinants of health, such as poverty and discrimination.
- Legislation provides the authority and tools necessary to respond to public health emergencies, such as pandemics or natural disasters. It allows governments to allocate resources, implement containment measures, and coordinate responses among various agencies and jurisdictions.
- Legislation has been instrumental in reducing tobacco use and curbing substance abuse. Laws restricting tobacco sales, advertising, and public smoking have contributed to significant reductions in smoking rates. Similarly, regulations on alcohol and drug sales help prevent substance abuse.
- Legislation can prohibit or regulate harmful practices that affect population health, such as the sale of unsafe products, deceptive marketing of health-related products, or predatory lending practices that impact social determinants of health.
- Legislation can expand access to healthcare services through measures like the Affordable Care Act (ACA) in the United States or similar laws in other countries. These laws may require insurance coverage, expand Medicaid, or create health insurance marketplaces, making healthcare services more accessible to populations.

Laws

- Laws can stress immunizations and preventive services, ensuring that a significant portion of the population is protected against vaccine-preventable diseases. These measures help establish and maintain herd immunity, reducing the spread of infectious diseases.
- Environmental laws and regulations are essential for protecting the health of populations. These laws set limits on pollution, hazardous substances, and

exposure to toxins, helping to prevent environmental health hazards that can lead to diseases and chronic conditions.

- Laws and regulations govern food safety standards, labeling, and nutritional content. These regulations help ensure that the food supply is safe and that consumers have access to accurate information about the foods consumed, promoting healthier diets and reducing foodborne illnesses.
- Laws can support public health education campaigns by allocating funding, mandating curriculum requirements, or regulating advertising and marketing practices related to health products and services.

Examples of Legislation

An example of legislation is Assembly Bill, A.B. 748 in California that requires every school to prominently display culturally appropriate and relevant mental health educational materials in areas frequented by school children grades 6–12. The materials describe common behaviors of those struggling with mental health and provide school-based contact information for resources, contact information for community resources, crisis intervention resources, and positive coping strategies (Robert Wood Johnson Foundation, n.d.-a). Go to the website for more information on AB-748 Pupil mental health.

Another example of legislation is Senate Bill, S.B. 1376 relating to Arizona's health curriculum in schools requires developmentally appropriate mental health instruction, including education on the impacts of mental health on overall physical health and social and emotional learning and also offers a consultation with mental health experts and mental health advocacy organizations. Navigate to the website to read about Senate Bill 1376.

A.B. 748 Pupil Mental Health: Mental Health Assistance Posters

Use the following resource to read about AB-748 in California.

https://leginfo.legislature.ca.gov/faces/billTextClient.xhtml?bill_id=202120220AB748

Senate Bill 1376

Use the following source to read the text of S.B. 1376 in Arizona.

https://www.azleg.gov/legtext/55leg/1R/bills/SB1376S.pdf

Secondary Prevention

Secondary prevention does not prevent disease, illness, or injury but promotes early detection through screening. Early detection improves the chance for positive health outcomes through addressing underlying causes, providing timely treatment, and limiting disability. Common pediatric secondary prevention interventions include assessing body mass index, testing vision and hearing, and screening for child maltreatment and developmental concerns. The benefits of secondary prevention for children are numerous and can have long-lasting positive effects on children's overall health status (Institute for Work and Health, 2015).

Secondary Prevention Examples

Demonstrating the effectiveness of secondary prevention through examples can build trust in public health interventions. It shows that proactive measures focus on early detection and intervention, aiming to minimize the impact of existing conditions, which can lead to greater support for such initiatives. In the following material, find several examples of secondary prevention to expand an understanding of population health.

Mental Health

Access to well visits are critical to a healthy developing child. Buka et al.'s (2022) article "The Family is the Patient: Promoting Early Childhood Mental Health in Pediatric Care" provides a strategy to holistically address mental health and identify risks early in the child's life. Mental health professionals are sometimes introduced into a children's life too late and only after problems have been established.

The strategy posed in by Buka et al. (2022) supports a system that advocates for healthy family environments, fosters parent–child and family relationships, explores parents' emotional and behavioral health, and takes a proactive, trauma-informed stance to integrate mental and physical healthcare with social support services. The core principles and priorities to this strategy include:

- Child/emotional behavioral health depends on the family environment.
- Healthy family environments come from healthy early relationships.
- Trauma-informed care promotes health and wellbeing of children and families.
- Integrating mental health and social health services within the primary care setting can advance child and family health.
- The primary focus should be on relationships.

In the textbox, navigate to the website for an article about The Family is the Patient: Promoting Early Childhood Mental Health in Pediatric Care (Buka et al., 2022).

The Family is the Patient: Promoting Early Childhood Mental Health in Pediatric Care

Read the following article to explore example programs promoting early childhood mental health.

https://doi.org/10.1542/peds.2021-053509L

A critical access point of addressing mental health for children has been identified in schools across the nation, especially for children from underserved backgrounds, children of color, children living in poverty, and children with disabilities. Examples of such strategies have been highlighted through legislative requirements improving mental health screenings and treatments as well as increasing staff knowledge and capacity.

- H.B. 1508 in Virginia requires schools to increase the number of full-time school counselors available to children.
- S.B. 5030 in Washington requires public schools to create and implement comprehensive counseling services, including identifying needs and an annual review process.
- S. 197 in Vermont provides financial backing for the development of a 2-year after-school program in underserved communities focusing on mental health and wellness as well as expanding school-based counseling services.

The textbox has a link with more information about secondary prevention mental health supports.

An Act Relating to the Provision of Mental Health Supports
Use the following resource to explore Vermont's S. 197.

https://legislature.vermont.gov/Documents/2022/Docs/ACTS/ACT112/ACT112%20As%20Enacted.pdf

States Recognized for Medicaid Program Innovations

The Arizona Health Care Cost Containment System (AHCCCS; n.d.) developed the Whole Person Care Initiative, a program to address SDOH, which offers a range of support services that includes referrals for transitional housing, transportation to community-based services (e.g., employment and food aid), and long-term care services to reduce social isolation. The following textbox includes a link to a whole person care initiative.

AHCCCS Whole Person Care Initiative (WPCI)
The program has shown reductions in emergency department visits by 31% and inpatient hospital stays by 44% as well as connecting the community to health providers across the state, which address physical and behavioral health.

https://www.azahcccs.gov/AHCCCS/Initiatives/AHCCCSWPCI/

California introduced a person-centered initiative to better serve homeless and unhoused communities, people who have been convicted of crimes, children with complex medical conditions, and aging communities. This model program provides coordinated and equitable care, connecting vulnerable populations to community resources for social, medical, and dental needs while strengthening the behavioral healthcare continuum. The textbox includes a link to information about California's journey to better health for all.

CalAIM: California's Opportunity to Transform Medi-Cal

Use the following resource to learn more about efforts to transform healthcare delivery.

https://www.dhcs.ca.gov/calaim

Paving the Road to Good Health Strategies for Increasing Medicaid Adolescent Well-Care Visits

https://www.medicaid.gov/sites/default/files/2019-12/paving-the-road-to-good-health.pdf

Adolescent Health Resources

Learn more about the Mount Sanai Adolescent Health Center.

https://www.mountsinai.org/locations/adolescent-health-center

Adolescent-Centered Care

Adolescence can be a period of significant risk-taking behaviors, and children living in underserved areas are particularly vulnerable given the lack of support resources and the complex role that Adverse Childhood Experiences (ACEs) play in adolescent decision making. The absence of accessible mental health services, extracurricular activities, and positive role models can exacerbate the challenges faced by these youth. ACEs, such as trauma, neglect, or household dysfunction, can significantly impact adolescents decision-making processes, often leading to engagement in risky behaviors as a way to cope or find temporary relief from emotional pain. To address this vulnerability, it is essential to prioritize targeted interventions and support systems in underserved communities, offering not only resources but also fostering resilience, empowerment, and opportunities for positive development. By recognizing and addressing these unique challenges, healthcare professionals can strive to create a safer and more supportive environment for adolescents in underserved areas, ultimately reducing the risks associated with this critical stage of life Centers for Disease Control and Prevention, (2021).

The Centers for Medicaid Services (2014) released a report with strategies to increase engagement in well-care visit strategies to promote more time spent with dedicated healthcare providers. Also identified were potential risks to intervene with supportive strategies and resources that can influence the physical, psychological, emotional, social, and mental health of an adolescent.

The Mount Sinai Adolescent Health Center, based in the East Harlem neighborhood of New York City, provides free comprehensive primary care, mental health counseling and resources, sexual health, and nutrition and wellness programs. The health center "support a diverse population of at-risk children, adolescents, and young adults (ages 10 through 26)," and on average in a year "serve more than 12,000 patients, who log more than 50,000 visits" (Mount Sinai Adolescent Health Center, n.d., para. 1). This health center helps overcome barriers of adolescence healthcare needs by (a) providing services that are free, confidential, and within proximity to public transportation; (b) allowing for flexible walk-in appointments with evening and weekend hours; and (c) maintaining a diverse staff that is representative in terms of race/ethnicity and primary language used. The textbox includes a link to Mount Sanai Adolescent Health Center.

Physical/Social/Emotional Health

A 2019 article by Walker et al. discusses the Juntos for Better Health Project, a project that focuses on creating access to prevention and treatment options for diabetes, depression, and obesity. The project is made up of a team of health professionals who set up clinics in available spaces within communities, such as libraries and employee break rooms and kitchens. This model dates to the late 1800s, when public health nursing was rooted in civic and church organizations. This program targets an underserved area of South Texas were 94.6% of the residents are Latino and suffer from poverty, lower education levels, transportation barriers, and inadequate access to healthcare. The mobile healthcare team consists of a qualified mental health professional (MHP), medical assistant (MA), family nurse practitioner (FNP) or physician assistant (PA), and a community health worker (CHW) serving as a patient navigator. The team performs intake information, vital signs, medical history, physical health assessment, mental health assessment, and exit interviews with referrals to medical facilities.

Go to the textbox to discover how the mobile traveling health care team reaches clients experiencing disparities in healthcare access.

Mobile Traveling Healthcare Teams: An Innovative Delivery System for Underserved Populations

Read the full article to learn more about the Juntos for Better Health Project.

https://ojin.nursingworld.org/table-of-contents/volume-23-2018/number-3-september-2018/mobile-traveling-healthcare-teams/

The CDC (2018b) offers a comprehensive registry of programs that have been effective in reducing risk behaviors in young people. Example strategies addressed by these programs include:

- HIV/AIDS prevention
- sexually transmitted infection (STI) prevention
- substance abuse prevention
- school dropout and failure prevention
- personal and social development
- cognitive development
- social and emotional development and life skills development
- protective factors against pregnancy and sexual victimization
- bullying prevention
- obesity support
- depression and anxiety support
- mental health assessments

In the textbox, learn more about how several federal agencies have identified youth-related programs that focus on a variety of health topics, risk behaviors and the settings.

Registries of Programs Effective in Reducing Youth Risk Behaviors

A variety of federal agencies have youth-related programs that focus on important health topics, such as risky behaviors and the settings. Each agency listed has its own method and criteria for offering the programs. To learn more, explore the website.

https://www.cdc.gov/healthyyouth/adolescenthealth/registries.htm

A description of the Trevor Project, found in the textbox provides 24/7 support for the lesbian, gay, bisexual, transgender, queer, intersex, asexual, and more (LGBTQIA+) youth community, connecting individuals with counselors, supplying tools to help someone else, offering comprehensive research for educational topics, and providing opportunities to join a community of loving and supporting individuals.

The Trevor Project

Explore the Trevor Project website for more information on resources and support for LGBTQIA+ young people.

www.trevorproject.org

Implicit or explicit forms of harassment or discrimination have become pervasive in the LGBTQIA+ community and affect the psychological health of those abused by micro aggressions, threats, or violence. Gender-based harassment includes behaviors that can harmfully reinforce societal gender norms, perpetuate stereotypes, and disrespect or discriminate against a person based on sex, gender identity, or sexual orientation. The information found in the textbox stresses AAP's call to attention to this societal problem to reinforce work and learning environments that support pediatric physicians in the delivery of inclusive and supportive healthcare to vulnerable youth in the LGBTQIA+ community.

Creating Work and Learning Environments Free of Gender-Based Harassment in Pediatric Health Care

The following report by Byerley et al. (2022) clearly outlines the AAP position statement as well as recommendations of how to support a zero-tolerance environment.

https://publications.aap.org/pediatrics/article/150/3/e2022058880/188902/Creating-Work-and-Learning-Environments-Free-of?autologincheck=redirected

Maternal and Child Health

For decades, home visits during pregnancy and early in the life of a child have shown positive outcomes to improve the lives of children and families. Home visits during pregnancy and in the early life of a child are a preventive healthcare strategy aimed at providing support, education, and healthcare services to expectant mothers and families with young children in the comfort of home. These visits are typically conducted by trained healthcare professionals or home visitors. Positive health outcomes associated with home visits during pregnancy and early childhood include improved prenatal care, healthier pregnancy outcomes, enhancing parenting bonding and skills, improved maternal mental health, positive infant health and development, increased breastfeeding rates, reduction in childhood injuries, early detection related to health and psychosocial issues, increased immunization rates, greater access to community resources, greater health equity and reduced disparities and overall family wellbeing (Health Resources and Services Administration, 2022).

The HRSA Maternal, Infant, And Early Childhood Home Visiting Program reduces childhood abuse and neglect, supports positive parenting strategies, addresses maternal and child health, promotes child development, and prepares children for school. Home visitors meet regularly with families and teach parenting skills communication strategies; screen for postpartum depression, substance use, and violence; screen children for autism and other developmental disabilities; and connect the families with resources to address any unmet needs. Learn more by going to the website in the textbox.

The Maternal, Infant, and Early Childhood Home Visiting Program
Read the 2023 HRSA brief.

https://mchb.hrsa.gov/sites/default/files/mchb/about-us/program-brief.pdf

North Carolina developed a maternal/perinatal telehealth policy during the COVID-19 pandemic that provided telehealth and home visit care to patients: provided reimbursement to perinatal providers for remote blood pressure monitoring, physiological monitoring, and lactation services; and conducted postpartum depression screenings by video, phone, and online portal messaging. Read the North Carolina maternal/perinatal telehealth policy on the following page.

Environmental Health

A 2016 article by Gratale and Haushalter describes the Nemours Children's Health System initiative, which encompasses the navigator model, made up of community health workers who work with children and families to identify environmental factors in home environments and educate families on how to eliminate or reduce factors to avoid asthma attacks. Community Health Workers also work with the Nemours Children's Health System care coordinators and community partners to connect families to social services, such as housing, childcare, and food. Through this initiative, Nemours Children's Health System works across sectors, including public health, housing, childcare, and other sectors that can positively influence the places children live, learn, and play. Additionally, Nemours Children's Health System works in community advocacy through public health campaigns like educating the schools on the dangers of bus idling that can worsen childhood asthma (Gratale & Haushalter, 2016).

The National Academy of Medicine model is replicable across the United States to address other environmental-related diseases, like lead poisoning, cancer prevention from plastics, pesticide exposures in rural America, and pediatric behavioral health and childhood trauma.

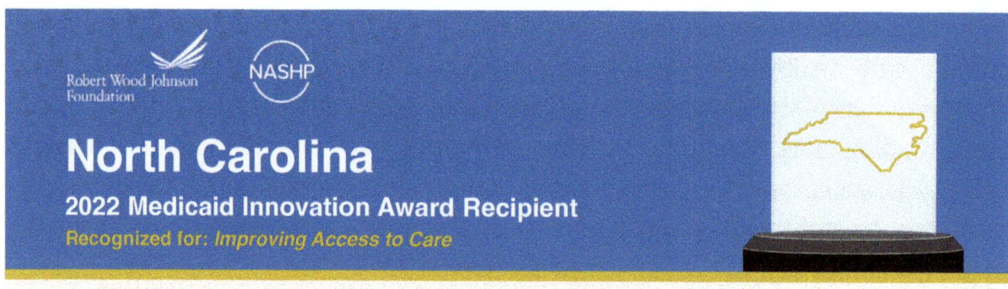

The Robert Wood Johnson Foundation (RWJF) and the National Academy for State Health Policy (NASHP) created the Medicaid Innovation Award to recognize states that implemented or enhanced initiatives to improve the lives of Medicaid enrollees and advance health equity, despite a sustained period of significant public health challenges. Selected by a panel of expert advisers, awards were given in six categories: (1) Enrollment Innovations, (2) Improving Access to Care, (3) Initiatives to Address Social Determinants of Health, (4) Care Coordination Initiatives for Vulnerable Populations, (5) Initiatives to Address Health Disparities, and (6) Promising or Emerging Initiatives.

North Carolina developed a comprehensive approach for pre- and postnatal care during the COVID-19 pandemic, including broad telehealth capabilities.

North Carolina Medicaid Fast Facts

27% of North Carolina residents are covered by Medicaid	More than 55% of births are covered by Medicaid in North Carolina	60% of Medicaid enrollees in North Carolina are people of color

The Challenge

The perinatal period—from the beginning of pregnancy through one-year postpartum—is a critical period for the health of pregnant women and babies. When the COVID-19 pandemic hit, North Carolina's Medicaid agency was concerned that pregnant enrollees would not be able to access the screenings and ongoing care they need, which could lead to poorer health outcomes for moms and babies.

The Solution

North Carolina's Medicaid agency implemented a temporary maternal and perinatal telehealth policy in April 2020 to provide a broad range of care to individuals in their homes, ensuring pregnant enrollees received needed care. The policy included:

- **Telehealth care** for both new and established pregnant and postpartum patients
- **Telephone and online portal messaging** for established patients
- **Remote blood pressure, heart rate, and temperature monitoring** medical equipment
- **Pharmacy benefits**, including a three-month supply of needed medications and delivery directly to homes
- **Hybrid comprehensive telemedicine/home visits**
- **Postpartum depression screenings** conducted via video visit, telephone, or online patient portal messaging
- **Telehealth lactation services**

The Environmental Health Program at Children's Mercy in Kansas City, Missouri, is a nationally recognized program that includes a Pediatric Environmental Health Services Unit, a Healthy Homes Program, and a Healthy Schools and Childcare Program. They provide indoor and outdoor environmental assessments and health consulting and collaborate with communities and families to educate and advocate for better living environments. Navigate to the textbox to learn more about this environmental health program.

Robert Wood Johnson Foundation/NASHP, "North Carolina 2022 Medicaid Innovation Award Recipient," p. 1.

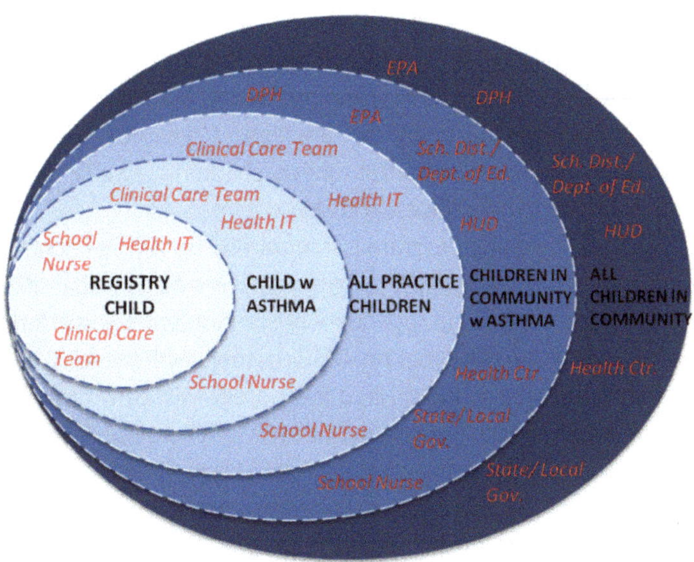

Figure 3.1 The National Academy of Medicine Model. Nemours's nested model beings with children who have been placed on Nemours's asthma registries and extends out to all children in the six targeted communities. Note: Black text = target population; red text = interventions.

Environmental health and lead poisoning in children are critically important topics that intersect at the nexus of public health, child development, and environmental science. Environmental health focuses on the prevention of diseases and injuries that result from environmental factors. It encompasses a broad range of concerns, including air and water quality, food safety, chemical exposures, and more. By addressing these factors, environmental health safeguards the wellbeing of individuals and communities. Lead is a neurotoxin, and children are particularly susceptible to its effects. Even low levels of lead exposure can harm a child's developing brain, leading to cognitive deficits, learning disabilities, and behavioral problems.

Environmental Health Program

Learn more about these comprehensive offerings from Children's Mercy in Kansas City.

https://www.childrensmercy.org/in-the-community/community-programs-with-childrens-mercy/environmental-health-program/

Nursing College Collaborates with the Douglas County Health Department

Dr. Kiley Petersmith, director of the Center for Diversity and Community Engagement at NMC, in partnership with the Douglas County Health Department (DCHD), offers point-of-care lead and hemoglobin testing for children under the age of 7 in the Omaha/Council Bluffs metropolitan area in an effort to prevent childhood lead exposure and poisoning. Lead poisoning remains a critical concern for infants, toddlers, and preschoolers residing in Douglas County in Omaha, Nebraska. Lead exposure can cause permanent damage to a child's developing brain, as well as other organs. The damage may be irreversible.

Omaha is one of the nation's largest federally superfund sites, increasing the risk of exposure to children in Douglas County. Compounding the dangers of environmental contamination, SDOH such as poverty, food insecurity, old housing stock, historical redlining, and difficulty accessing healthcare are highest in number within this county's zip codes. Lead exposure also comes from paint, children's jewelry, imported goods (including canned food), candy, spices, and skin creams.

Information for Health Care Professionals

Click into the link to learn more about the Douglas County Health lead poisoning prevention initiative.

https://www.douglascountyhealth.com/lead-poisoning-prevention/27-lead-poisoning-prevention/632-information-for-health-professionals

The screening program is integrated into NMC's Bachelor Degree of Science in Nursing (BSN) program to serve as a clinical site where students are engaged in secondary prevention screening efforts within the community. In this program, NMC partners with the local health department and area schools, Head Start programs, early childhood learning classrooms, and daycare facilities to offer point-of-care lead testing within the community where children learn and play. Registered nurses (RNs) in the program work with health department leaders, teachers, and other nurses in these childhood program systems to educate parents on the existing dangers of lead exposure, as well as obtain consent to perform the screenings.

Laboratory results are received in real time and reported directly to parents and DCHD. Furthermore, the screenings are at no cost to the children or families. Resources are provided during the screenings to connect those who are identified as having exposure to lead with further resources, environmental assessments, and environmental mitigation. Learn more about Douglas County Health Department superfund site and childhood lead program.

Tertiary Prevention

Tertiary prevention refers to interventions that manage chronic disease complications and worsening of the individual's condition. Tertiary prevention also has aspects of health promotion and provides education and treatment to help individuals manage long-term, complex health problems and injuries to positively affect function and maintain/improve quality of life. In the pediatric population, tertiary prevention measures are appropriate for children with diabetes mellitus, traumatic injury/harm, depression, and other long-term complex conditions (Institute for Work and Health, 2015). There are three elements to health promotion found in tertiary care: good governance for health, health literacy, and healthy cities.

Good Governance for Health

One of the roles of U.S. government is to support the health and wellbeing of all citizens through services and policies that promote the attainment of health. All branches of government—legislative, executive, and judicial—share in this responsibility. Governmental policymakers establish health policies. The goal of any health policy should be preventing citizens from becoming ill or injured (WHO, 2016). National and state examples may include taxes on unhealthy or potentially harmful products (e.g., tobacco and alcohol), seat belt or child car seat laws, and emission limits to reduce air and water pollution.

Health Literacy

Autonomous decision making is important to attaining health for an individual. For autonomy to exist, individuals need to have the knowledge and skills to make healthy lifestyle choices. Health literacy is a cornerstone of autonomous decision making. Healthy People 2030 (Office of Disease Prevention and Health Promotion, n.d.-a) has updated the definition of health literacy to reflect its central focus in attainment of health. According to Healthy People 2030, **health literacy** is "the degree to which individuals have the ability to find, understand, and use information and services to inform health-related decisions and actions for themselves and others" (Office of Disease Prevention and Health Promotion, n.d.-a, "How Does?" section). Healthcare organizations contribute to health literacy through availability of educational resources written with the public in mind to aid in educating and promoting decision making. When caring for pediatric patients, it is important to assess the health literacy of parents and caregivers, navigate to the textbox for more information.

Healthy People 2030

Learn about health literacy, a main goal for Healthy People 2030.

https://youtu.be/BG-iY-em7mk

Healthy Cities

City leaders are instrumental in creating and sustaining a strong infrastructure that supports the health of its citizens. Community government and planning commissions have a role in terms of creating city walking paths, public health departments, or community-based programs that promote health. A healthy city is on a path of continuous quality improvement in terms of physical and social structures that enable citizens to engage in healthful behaviors (WHO, 2016). Healthy cities strategically address violence, food deserts, and lack of access to healthcare to promote the wellbeing of the community.

Tertiary Prevention Examples

Examples of tertiary care resources are essential for various stakeholders, including children, parents, caregivers healthcare professionals, policymakers, researchers, and the public. These resources serve as valuable tools for education, decision-making, quality improvement, research, and advocacy, ultimately contributing to better healthcare outcomes and a more informed and empowered healthcare community.

Children's Hospital and Medical Center's Complex Care Clinic

Learn more about the Children's Hospital and Medical Center's Complex Care Clinic.

https://www.childrensomaha.org/department/complex-care-clinic/

National Center for Children in Poverty

Learn more about the National Center for Children in Poverty on this website.

https://www.nccp.org

Wide-Reaching Resources

The Children's Hospital and Medical Center's Complex Care Clinic in Omaha, Nebraska, uses a family-centered team approach to helping children with complex medical conditions. More information about the clinic, found in the textbox provides material on an initial assessment, ongoing consultation, delivery of healthcare services, medical case management, and the evaluation of children with a variety of developmental disabilities.

The National Center for Children in Poverty moves research into action to improve the lives of children, make meaningful change, and decrease the number of families experiencing hardship. Low-income families and children benefit from this ongoing work. This team delivers the research to important constituents, child advocates, and policymakers to create effective policies that promote healthy child development and form strong families. Navigate to the National Center for Children in Poverty using the link found in the textbox.

Babies

Babies are an essential part of the movement toward health equity because due to the position as identified as earliest stage of life. Ensuring equitable access to quality healthcare and supportive environments for infants is crucial in breaking the cycle of health disparities that can persist throughout a person's life. By addressing the health needs of babies and families, healthcare providers have an opportunity to lay a foundation for lifelong wellbeing and reduce health inequalities from the very beginning of life. Promoting health equity for babies is not only a matter of social justice but also an investment in a healthier and more equitable future for all.

The March of Dimes (n.d.) initiated a movement toward health equity, "opening the door for all moms to have access to care and protecting the health of families by advocating for their rights." See more information about the March of Dimes in the textbox.

Chronic Conditions or Disabilities

A diverse population includes children with chronic conditions or disabilities (different abilities) who have a wide variety of life experiences. These children live and play in every community. The degree to which these children can perform and fully participate in a realistic lifestyle and lead fulfilling lives is contingent on what kind of quality accommodations and resources are received. Chronic conditions or disabilities in children refer to conditions or impairments that affect a child's physical, cognitive, sensory, emotional, or social abilities and may impact overall development and daily functioning. These chronic conditions or disabilities in children can vary widely in the nature, severity, age of onset, and holistic health care management.

A population health framework for at-risk children is an era where the overall health of a community is recognized as crucial, focusing on children's wellbeing is a fundamental aspect. Population health provides a comprehensive framework for understanding and addressing the health of not just individuals but entire groups of children who may be at risk of developing various medical, emotional, or psychosocial conditions. By considering all of the factors that influence children's health within communities, healthcare providers can create targeted interventions to promote healthier outcomes and reduce risks.

Children with chronic conditions or disabilities represent a significant challenge in the realm of pediatric healthcare. Conditions such as diabetes, asthma, or congenital heart defects require specialized care and attention throughout a child's life. Managing children's chronic conditions or disabilities involves a complex interplay of medical, psychological, and social factors including comprehensive healthcare services, rehabilitation programs, and support networks. Understanding the nuances of these conditions in children is essential for healthcare providers, parents, caregivers, and communities to provide optimal care to help children lead fulfilling lives.

A Mother of a Movement

Read about the March for Babies movement.

https://www.marchforbabies.org/Registration/ads-signup?utm_source=google&utm_medium=cpc&utm_campaign=2023mfb&utm_content=brand&bt=google&gclid=CjwKCAiAu5agBhBzEiwAdiR5tFZYZFPE6y1wGxTLqT4VpUrzGVAgyKhc4ksMCsYRRbN3EHqtvPv-mhoCgq4QAvD_BwE&gclsrc=aw.ds

List of Chronic Conditions or Disabilities

Physical:

Cerebral Palsy is a group of movement disorders caused by damage to the brain, affecting muscle control and coordination.

Spina Bifida is a neural tube defect that can lead to varying degrees of paralysis and other physical challenges.

Muscular Dystrophy is a group of genetic disorders that cause progressive muscle weakness and degeneration.

Juvenile Diabetes (JD Type 1 diabetes) is a chronic medical condition characterized by the body's inability to produce insulin, a hormone necessary for regulating blood sugar (glucose) levels.

Asthma is a chronic respiratory condition that affects the airways in the lungs. It causes airways to become inflamed and narrowed, leading to a variety of symptoms, including difficulty breathing, wheezing, coughing, and chest tightness. Asthma can vary in severity from mild to severe.

Congenital Heart Defect (CHD) is a congenital heart anomaly or congenital heart disease, described as a structural abnormality in the heart or the large blood vessels near the heart that is present at birth. A variety of defects can vary in complexity and severity, and may affect the heart's walls, valves, arteries, veins, or chambers. CHDs are the most common type of birth defects, and can occur in isolation or as part of a more complex syndrome.

Cystic Fibrosis (CF) is a genetic, inherited disorder that primarily affects the respiratory and digestive systems. It is caused by mutations in the CFTR (cystic fibrosis transmembrane conductance regulator) gene, which leads to the production of thick and sticky mucus in various organs, including the lungs, pancreas, liver, and intestines. The accumulation of this mucus can result in a wide range of health problems.

- Intellectual:

  An Intellectual disability is characterized by limitations in intellectual functioning (such as reasoning, learning, and problem-solving) and adaptive behaviors, often with an onset before the age of 18.

  Down Syndrome is a genetic condition caused by an extra chromosome 21, leading to cognitive impairments and physical features like distinctive facial characteristics.

- Sensory:

  Visual impairment is a condition that results in partial or complete loss of vision, such as congenital blindness or visual impairment due to disease or injury.

  Hearing impairment is hearing loss which can be congenital or acquired and ranges from mild to profound.

- Communication:

  Speech-language disorders are conditions that affect children's ability to communicate effectively, such as stuttering, speech sound disorders, or language disorders.

  Autism Spectrum Disorder (ASD) is a developmental disorder characterized by challenges in social communication, repetitive behaviors, and a range of strengths and difficulties in various areas of functioning.

- Emotional and Behavioral:

  Attention-Deficit/Hyperactivity Disorder (ADHD) is a neurodevelopmental disorder characterized by inattention, hyperactivity, and impulsivity.

Anxiety Disorder is a condition such as generalized anxiety disorder or social anxiety disorder that can significantly impact a child's emotional wellbeing.

- Neurological:

  Epilepsy is a condition characterized by recurrent seizures due to abnormal electrical activity in the brain.

  Tourette Syndrome is a neurological disorder characterized by repetitive, involuntary movements and vocalizations (tics).

- Developmental: developmental delays impact children's ability to reach developmental milestones (e.g., motor skills, language development) that may indicate another underlying condition or disability.

Adapted from Ward & Hisley, 2016.

Several resources are available for children with chronic conditions or disabilities. The United Nations International Children's Emergency Fund (UNICEF) organization or now called the United Nations Children's Fund is a good example of "every child has the right to live in an inclusive world," see textbox for details information and resources.

Children with Disabilities

Visit this UNICEF webpage to learn more about children with disabilities and access to featured resources.

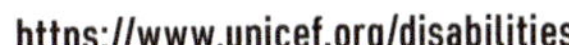
https://www.unicef.org/disabilities

Did you know many school-aged children and adolescents have at least one chronic health condition, such as asthma, obesity, and/or behavior/learning problems? The healthcare needs of children with chronic illness can be complex and continuous. These conditions include both daily management and addressing potential emergencies (CDC, 2017). The textbox provides recommendations for caring for managing chronic health conditions.

CDC Healthy Schools, Managing Chronic Health Conditions

The following CDC webpage provides an overview of chronic health conditions in school-aged children.

https://www.cdc.gov/healthyschools/chronicconditions.htm

Founded in 1970, the Juvenile Diabetes Research Foundation (JDRF; n.d.) "is the leading global organization harnessing the power of research, advocacy, and community engagement to advance life-changing breakthroughs for type 1 diabetes." The textbox has more information about the JDRF.

Juvenile Diabetes Research Foundation
Learn more about the JDRF by exploring this website.
https://www.jdrf.org

The American Academy of Allergy, Asthma, and Immunology website provides an overview of asthma symptoms and diagnosis. Conditions and treatments include a variety of up-to-date links with additional information. The material in the website also includes information for allergists and the public.

American Academy of Allergy, Asthma, and Immunology
Learn more about asthma symptoms, diagnosis, and treatment.
https://www.aaaai.org/Conditions-Treatments/asthma

The National Environmental Education Foundation Environmental (NEEF; n.d.) works in partnership with the CDC's National Asthma Control Program: "NEEF's Environmental Management of Pediatric Asthma Guidelines training equips pediatric healthcare providers and clinicians with knowledge and tools to manage environmental asthma triggers and intervention strategies." See the textbox to learn more detailed information about this agency.

National Environmental Education Foundation
Learn more about the National Environmental Education Foundation and pediatric asthma.
https://www.neefusa.org/health/asthma

The Children's Heart Foundation funds congenital heart defect (CHD) initiatives. The vision promotes the worldwide idea that every child born with a congenital heart defect has the chance to live a long, healthy life. Video clips, inspirational stories, and facts about genetics and causes showcase needed information about this chronic condition are found in the textbox.

The Children's Heart Foundation
Learn more about congenital heart defects on the Children's Heart Foundation website.
https://www.childrensheartfoundation.org

Cystic fibrosis is an inherited disease that causes severe damage to the lungs, digestive system, and other body organs. The Mayo Clinic website in the textbox provides current information on signs and symptoms, when to see a doctor, risk factors, complications, and prevention strategies (Chalmers, n.d.).

Mayo Foundation for Medical Education and Research
See the Mayo Clinic webpage on Cystic Fibrosis to learn more.
https://www.mayoclinic.org/diseases-conditions/cystic-fibrosis/symptoms-causes/syc-20353700

The Epilepsy Foundation's (n.d.) mission is "to lead the fight to overcome the challenges of living with epilepsy and to accelerate therapies to stop seizures, find cures, and save lives". The Epilepsy Foundation website has information on finding local support, upcoming events, and resources. Current news articles and stories provide compelling information about this chronic condition. Research and innovations investigate important topics to establish facts, reach reliable conclusions, and propel advancements. Navigate to the textbox to better understand Epilepsy.

Epilepsy Foundation
Learn more about the Epilepsy Foundation's efforts on this website.
https://www.epilepsy.com

Summary

In summary, after reading Section 3, learners now have an appreciation for population health as a vital framework for understanding and improving the health of children within a community. This section discusses, population health an approach that considers the health of an entire community or population, rather than focusing solely on individual health. It emphasizes the social determinants of health that influence children's wellbeing. The health of children and its intricate link to the health of communities is discussed. At the primary prevention level, emphasis is placed on strategies aimed at preventing health problems before occurrence. Secondary prevention focuses on early detection and intervention to mitigate the progression of health issues. The tertiary prevention information involves managing and reducing the impact of established health conditions in children. Furthermore, Section 3 provides valuable insights into locating resources that support population health efforts, ultimately contributing to improvement in overall health outcomes for children. After reading Section 3, learners have a better understanding of the intricacies of a population health framework, levels of prevention and health promotion along with guidance in finding accompanying resources in the context of pediatric care. Section 3 assists learners in the transition to Section 4 found on Cognella Active Learning that has interactive exercises, case studies, critical thinking exercises, Next Generation NCLEX style questions, and math questions.

Credit

Fig. 3.1: Danielle Gratale and Alisa Haushalter, "Optimizing Health Outcomes for Children with Asthma in Delaware: A Population Health Case Report," National Academy of Medicine Perspectives. Copyright © 2016 by National Academy of Sciences.

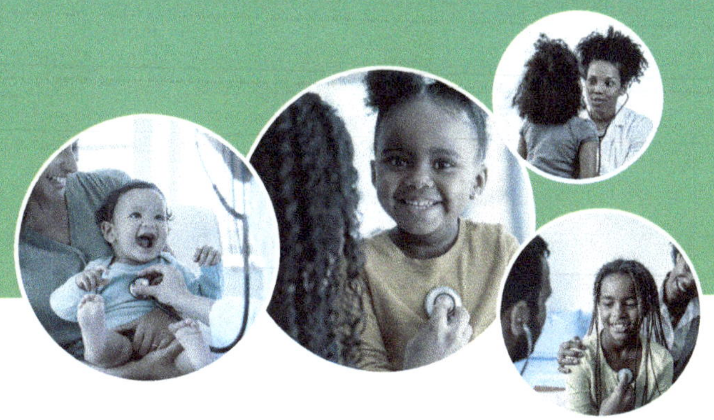

SECTION 4

Active Learning

Dr. Meg Blair and Dr. Susan Ward

Section 4 Introduction

Section 4 is found on Cognella Active Learning and contains interactive exercises, case studies, critical thinking exercises, NCLEX next-gen style questions, and math questions.

Book Summary

The Pediatric Population Health book allows readers to embark on a journey that explores the landscape of children's health and wellness. The book introduces population health as a framework for understanding primary care as it relates to health promotion. Public health surveillance and health policy enable the reader to discover a deeper understanding of the factors that influence children's health outcomes. A culture of health, rooted in sensitivity and respect for cultural differences, emerges as a pivotal concept, underscoring the need for culturally sensitivity care to ensure children of diverse backgrounds receive equitable access to health services. The emerging topic of functional medicine focuses on addressing the root causes of disease rather than just treating symptoms. The book's intent stresses a broader mission of fostering healthier communities through collaborative efforts and community-based education that empowers children, parents and caregivers. The critical role of social determinants of health is illuminated, showcasing how these factors profoundly impact children's wellbeing, from infancy through adolescence.

Readers explore children's growth and development, rooted in the framework of population health. The book illuminates the interconnectedness of children's well-being and the broader context of community health, offering a holistic perspective on the factors shaping children's lives. From infancy to adolescence, the book provides a good understanding of growth and development and milestones that contribute to children's overall health and wellbeing. The areas that shape children's health are physical growth and sensory development, gross motor skills, fine motor skills, psychosocial development, play, and communication. One of the book's important themes is the role of developmental screening in early identification of children at risk. A discussion of standard developmental theories sheds light on the influence that each theorists has on children's maturation: Ainsworth, Freud, Erikson, Piaget, Kohlberg, Gardner, and Fowler.

The book also offers a detailed approach to primary, secondary, and tertiary levels of prevention and health promotion, equipping readers with the knowledge and tools to promote and safeguard children's health at every stage of development. It also provides guidance on finding primary, secondary, and tertiary prevention resources, ensuring that communities have the necessary support systems to nurture the well-being of children and families.

Population Health as a Framework for Wellness in Children serves as a guide that not only explores the multifaceted world of children's health but also empowers children, families, communities, and policymakers to take proactive steps toward creating healthier, more equitable environments for children. With a focus on population health, public policy, cultural competence, and collaborative efforts, this book serves as a ray of hope for a future where all children have the opportunity to thrive and reach their fullest potential.

GLOSSARY

Anticipatory guidance: preemptive advice that addresses physical, emotional, psychological, and developmental changes for each age group. Providing information before the next stage of development assists caregivers in understanding the expected growth and developmental parameters.

Culture: based on racial, ethnic, linguistic, or geographical groups and also based on beliefs, values, customs, communication patterns, and ways of thinking (CDC, 2021).

Culture of Health: A culture of health is a concept developed by the Robert Wood Johnson Foundation, a prominent philanthropic organization dedicated to improving health and healthcare in the United States. It represents a vision for a society in which health and wellbeing are valued and promoted as shared priorities at all levels of society, and where individuals and communities have the resources and opportunities to make healthy choices (Robert Wood Johnson Foundation. n.d.-c;. Robert Wood Johnson Foundation. 2018)

Community-based participatory research: acknowledges community as a unit and builds on the strengths and resources existing within the community. This research builds a relationship and partnership that is collaborative and equitable and empowers the power-sharing process that tends to social inequities.

Cultural sensitivity: allows healthcare providers to understand the society in which an individual and population dwells.

Developmental screening: used in early identification of children at risk for cognitive, motor, communication, or social-emotional delays.

Developmental milestones: developmental milestones are behaviors or skills that illustrate a child's growth in several areas. The milestones have been established based on what most children can do at a certain age. These milestones are a set of functional skills or age-specific tasks that most children can do at a certain age range.

Discrimination: is the unjust or prejudicial treatment based on race, religion, age, gender or sexual orientation, disability/ability, and more (Davis, 2020). Discrimination occurs both individually and systemically. Examples of individual discrimination include slurs, micro aggressions, and violence.

Disease prevention: when an individual or a population addresses the risk factors associated with disease and minimizes the burden of disease (WHO, n.d.).

Growth spurts: create surges in growth in height and weight, are a normal part of children's development, and occur at different stages during childhood, until they reach physical maturity.

Gut microbiome: the collective genomes of microorganisms in the gut (Valdes et al., 2018).

Gut microbiota: the community of gut microorganisms themselves (Valdes et al., 2018).

Gut dysbiosis: imbalance of gut microbiota associated with an unhealthy outcome and can have a negative impact on neurocognitive development, including behavioral and mood problems (Slykerman et al., 2017).

Health equity: providing everyone with a fair opportunity to attain full health potential and ensuring no one is disadvantaged from achieving full potential due to social circumstances (Robert Wood Johnson Foundation, n.d.-a).

Health literacy: "the degree to which individuals have the ability to find, understand, and use information and services to inform health-related decisions and actions for themselves and others" (Office of Disease Prevention and Health Promotion, n.d.-a, "How Does?" section).

Object permanence: refers to the knowledge that objects and people continue to exist even when they cannot be sensed (seen or heard; Ansorge, 2020).

Population health: the Centers for Disease Control and Prevention (CDC, 2020a) views population health as an approach that allows health departments to interface with practice that create policy for change to happen locally. This approach uses many partnerships among different sectors of the community such as public health, industry, academia, healthcare, and local government entities.

Primary care: healthcare services that are accessible, community-based, person-centered, and achieve better health at lower costs (American Academy of Family Physicians, n.d.).

Primary prevention: focuses on prevention of the development of disease and illness and the prevention of injury. Primary prevention strategies promote the physical health of children as well as social and economic health.

Public health surveillance: the systematic and ongoing collection, analysis, and interpretation of health-related data (CDC, 2018a; Klaucke et al., 1988).

Secondary prevention: does not prevent disease, illness, or injury but promotes early detection through screening (Institute for Work and Health, 2015).

Social determinants of health (SDOH): the conditions in which people were born, live, learn, work, play, and pray (Office of Disease Prevention and Health Promotion, n.d.-b). The five key domains of SDOH from Healthy People 2030 include economic stability, education access and quality, healthcare access and quality, neighborhood and built environment, and social and community context.

Tertiary prevention: interventions that manage chronic disease complications and worsening of the individual's condition. Tertiary prevention also provides education and treatment to help individuals manage long-term, complex health problems and injuries to positively impact function and maintain/improve quality of life.

Vulnerable populations: have been identified through epidemiological studies as having poorer health outcomes. Vulnerable populations are also considered groups and communities at a higher risk for poor health as a result of the barriers they experience to social, economic, political, and environmental resources, as well as limitations due to illness or disability.

REFERENCES

Agency for Healthcare Research and Quality. (n.d.). *Health literacy universal precautions toolkit* (2nd ed.). https://www.ahrq.gov/health-literacy/improve/precautions/tool11.html

Ages and Stages Questionnaire. (n.d.). *Home*. https://agesandstages.com

Ainsworth, M. D. (1964). Patterns of attachment behavior shown by the infant in interaction with his mother. *Merrill-Palmer Quarterly of Behavior and Development, 10*(1), 51–58. http://www.jstor.org/stable/23082925

Alliance of Nurses for Healthy Environments. (n.d.). *Climate change & health*. https://envirn.org/climate-change/

American Academy of Allergy, Asthma, & Immunology. (n.d.). *Conditions and treatments*. https://www.aaaai.org/Conditions-Treatments

American Academy of Family Physicians (n.d.). *Primary care*. Retrieved July 21, 2023, from https://www.aafp.org/about/policies/all/primary-care.html

American Academy of Pediatrics. (n.d.-a). *Ages and stages*. https://www.healthychildren.org/English/ages-stages/Pages/default.aspx

American Academy of Pediatrics. (n.d.-b). *Baby*. https://www.healthychildren.org/English/ages-stages/baby/Pages/default.aspx

American Academy of Pediatrics. (n.d.-c). *Bright Futures*. https://brightfutures.aap.org/materials-and-tools/tool-and-resource-kit/Pages/Early-Childhood-Tools.aspx

American Academy of Pediatrics. (2022, February 2). *Social determinants of health screening resources*. https://www.aap.org/en/patient-care/screening-technical-assistance-and-resource-center/screening-resource-library/social-determinants-of-health/?page=1&sortDirection=1&sortField=Year

American Association of Colleges of Nursing. (n.d.). *Our initiatives*. https://www.aacnnursing.org/our-initiatives/education-practice/academic-practice-partnerships

American Association of Colleges of Nursing. (2021). *The essentials: Core competencies for professional nursing education*. https://www.aacnnursing.org/Essentials

American Nurses Association. (2016). *The nurse's role in ethics and human rights: Protecting and promoting individual worth, dignity, and human rights in practice settings*. https://www.nursingworld.org/~4af078/globalassets/docs/ana/ethics/ethics-and-human-rights-protecting-and-promoting-final-formatted-20161130.pdf

American Planning Association. (2022). *Fostering healthy communities through planning and public health collaboration*. https://planning-org-uploaded-media.s3.amazonaws.com/publication/download_pdf/Planning-Public-Health-Collaboration.pdf

American Public Health Association. (n.d.) *Racial equity & public health*. https://www.apha.org/-/media/Files/PDF/advocacy/SPEAK/210825_Racial_Equity_Fact_Sheet.ashx

Ansorge, R. (2020, August 17). *Piaget stages of development*. WebMD. https://www.webmd.com/children/piaget-stages-of-development

Arizona Health Care Costs Containment System. (n.d.). *AHCCCS whole person care initiative (WPCI)*. https://www.azahcccs.gov/AHCCCS/Initiatives/AHCCCSWPCI/

Armstrong, T. (2020, June 12). *The stages of faith according to James W. Fowler*. American Institute for Learning and Human Development. https://www.institute4learning.com/2020/06/12/the-stages-of-faith-according-to-james-w-fowler/

Bahadur, K., Pai, S., Thoby, E., & Petrova, A. (2018). Frequency of food insecurity and associated health outcomes in pediatric patients at a federally qualified health center. *Journal of Community Health, 43*, 896–900. https://doi.org/10.1007/s10900-018-0499-8

Barbero, C., Hafeedh Bin Abdullah, A., Wiggins, N., Garrettson, M., Jones, D., S. Guinn, A., Girod, C., Bradford, J., & Wennerstrom, A. (2022). Community health workers activities in public health programs to prevent violence: Coding roles and scope. *American Journal of Public Health, 112*(8), 1191–1201. https://doi.org/10.2105/AJPH.2022.306865

Bhattacharya, D., & Bhatt, J. (2017). Seven foundational principles of population health policy. *Population Health Management, 20*(5), 383–388. https://doi.org/10.1089/pop.2016.0148

Bradford, J., & Wennerstrom, A. (2022). Community health workers activities in public health programs to prevent violence: Coding roles and scope. *American Journal of Public Health, 112*(8), 1191–1201. https://doi.org/10.2105/AJPH.2022.306865

Build Healthy Places Network. (n.d.). *MeasureUp*. https://www.buildhealthyplaces.org/tools-resources/measure-up/

Buka, S. L., Beers, L. S., Biel, M. G., Counts, N. Z., Hudziak, J., Parade, S. H., Paris, R., Seifer, R., & Drury, S. S. (2022). The family is the patient: Promoting early childhood mental health in pediatric care. *Pediatrics, 149*(Suppl. 5), Article e2021053509L. https://doi.org/10.1542/peds.2021-053509l

Byerley, J. S., Dodson, N. A., St. Clair, T., & Walker, V. P. (2022). Creating work and learning environments free of gender-based harassment in pediatric healthcare. *Pediatrics, 150*(3), Article e2022058880. https://doi.org/10.1542/peds.2022-058880

Cartwright, K. (2001). Cognitive developmental theory and spiritual development. *Journal of Adult Development, 8*. https://doi.org/10.1023/A:1011386427919

Centers for Disease Control and Prevention (n.d.-a). *Milestone moments: Learn the signs. Act early.* https://www.cdc.gov/ncbddd/actearly/pdf/booklets/Milestone-Moments-Booklet21_Eng_Sng_FNL-508.pdf

Centers for Disease Control and Prevention. (n.d.-b). *National Notifiable Diseases Surveillance System (NNDSS)*. https://www.cdc.gov/nndss/index.html

Centers for Disease Control and Prevention (n.d.-c). *Prevention*. https://www.cdc.gov/pictureofamerica/pdfs/picture_of_america_prevention.pdf

Centers for Disease Control and Prevention. (2017). *Research brief: Chronic health conditions and academic achievement*. https://www.cdc.gov/healthyschools/chronic_conditions/pdfs/2017_02_15-CHC-and-Academic-Achievement_Final_508.pdf

Centers for Disease Control and Prevention. (2018a, November 15). *Introduction to public health surveillance*. https://www.cdc.gov/training/publichealth101/surveillance.html

Centers for Disease control and Prevention. (2018b, August 17). *Program registries*. https://www.cdc.gov/healthyyouth/adolescenthealth/registries.htm

Centers for Disease Control and Prevention (2018c, October 15). *The whole school, whole community, whole child (WSCC) model*. https://www.cdc.gov/healthyyouth/wscc/model.htm

Centers for Disease Control and Prevention (2020a). *Division of population health*. https://www.cdc.gov/populationhealth/index.html

Centers for Disease Control and Prevention. (2021, January 05). *Risk and protective factors*. https://www.cdc.gov/violenceprevention/aces/riskprotectivefactors.html

Centers for Disease Control and Prevention. (2022a, December 27). *Health literacy*. https://www.cdc.gov/healthliteracy/culture.html#:~:text=Culture%20can%20be%20defined%20by,behaving%20specific%20to%20a%20group

Centers for Disease Control and Prevention (2022b, December 29). *Milestones*. https://www.cdc.gov/ncbddd/actearly/milestones/index.html

Centers for Disease Control and Prevention (2022c). *National Center for Health Statistics*. https://www.cdc.gov/growthcharts/index.htm

Centers for Disease Control and Prevention. (2022d, December 08). *Social determinants of health at CDC*. https://www.cdc.gov/socialdeterminants/about.html

Centers for Medicare and Medicaid Services. (2014, February). *Paving the road to good health: Strategies for increasing Medicaid adolescent well-care visits*. U.S. Department of Health and Human Services. https://fhop.ucsf.edu/sites/fhop.ucsf.edu/files/custom_download/paving-the-road-to-good-health.pdf

Chalmers, S. (n.d.). *What is cystic fibrosis? A Mayo Clinic expert explains*. Mayo Clinic. https://www.mayoclinic.org/diseases-conditions/cystic-fibrosis/symptoms-causes/syc-20353700

Chandra, A., Acosta, J., Carman, K. G., Dubowitz, T., Leviton, L., Martin, L. T., Miller, C., Nelson, C., Orleans, T., Tait, M., Trujillo, M., Towe, V., Yeung, D., & Plough, A. L. (2017). Building a national culture of health: Background, action framework, measures, and next steps. *Rand Health Quarterly, 6*(2), 3. https://www.ncbi.nlm.nih.gov/pmc/articles/PMC5568157/

Cheney, C. (2022, February 16). *Quintuple aim: Health equity added to healthcare improvement directive*. HealthLeaders. https://www.healthleadersmedia.com/clinical-care/quintuple-aim-health-equity-added-healthcare-improvement-directive

Cherry, K. (2020, March 27). *Howard Gardner biography and theories*. Verywell Mind. https://www.verywellmind.com/howard-gardner-biography-2795511

Cherry, K. (2022a, November 14). *An overview of Sigmund Freud's theories*. Verywell Mind. https://www.verywellmind.com/freudian-theory-2795845

Cherry, K. (2022b, August 3). *Erik Erikson's stages of psychosocial development: A closer look at the eight psychological stages*. Verywell Mind. https://www.verywellmind.com/erik-eriksons-stages-of-psychosocial-development-2795740

Cherry, K. (2023, March 13). *7 main developmental theories: Child development theories of Freud, Erickson, and more*. Verywell Mind. https://www.verywellmind.com/child-development-theories-2795068

Children's Heart Foundation. (n.d.). *Home*. https://www.childrensheartfoundation.org

Chung, E. K., Siegel, B. S., Garg, A., Conroy, K., Gross, R. S., Long, D. A., Lewis, G., Osman, C. J., Messina, M. J., Wade, R., Yin, S., Cox, J., & Fiermam, A. H. (2016). Screening for social determinants of health among children and families living in poverty: A guide for clinicians. *Current Problems in Pediatric and Adolescent Healthcare, 46*(5), 135–153. http://doi.org/10.1016/j.cppeds.2016.02.004

Commonwealth of Massachusetts. (n.d.). *Department of Early Education and Care*. https://www.mass.gov/orgs/department-of-early-education-and-care

Conn, A. M., Szilagyi, M. A., Jee, S. H., Manly, J. T., Briggs, R., & Szilagyi, P. G. (2018). Parental perspectives of screening for adverse childhood experiences in pediatric primary care. *Families, Systems, & Health, 36*(1), 62–72. https://doi.org/10.1037/fsh0000311

Coveney, J., & O'Dwyer, L. (2009). Effects of mobility and location on food access. *Health & Place, 15*(1), 45–55. https://doi.org/10.1016/j.healthplace.2008.01.010

Davis, B. A. (2020, February 25). *Discrimination: A social determinant of health inequities*. HealthAffairs. https://www.healthaffairs.org/do/10.1377/forefront.20200220.518458/full/

de Goffau, M.C., Luopajärvi, K., Knip, M., Ilonen, J., Ruohtula, T., Härkönen, T., Orivuori, L., Hakala, S., Welling, G. W., Harmsen, H. J., & Vaarala, O. (2013). Fecal microbiota composition differs between children with β-cell autoimmunity and those without. *Diabetes, 62*(4), 1238–1244. https://doi.org/10.2337/db12-0526

Diversity Data Kids. (n.d.). *Child opportunity levels* [Map]. https://www.diversitydatakids.org/maps/

Environmental Health Sciences. (n.d.). *Environmental health news*. https://ehsciences.activehosted.com/index.php?action=social&chash=eddb904a6db773755d2857aacadb1cb0.1071&s=9df1945fd32f22cf4aa66b127ab23396

Environmental Protection Agency. (n.d.). *Environmental justice*. https://www.epa.gov/environmentaljustice

Epilepsy Foundation. (n.d.). *Home*. https://www.epilepsy.com

Fee, E. & Bu, Liping. (2011). The origins of public health nursing: The Henry Street Visiting Nurse Service. *American Journal of Public Health, 100*(7), 1206–1207. https://doi.org/10.2105/AJPH.2009.186049

Fowler, J., & Levin. R. (1984). Stages of faith: The psychology of human development and the quest for meaning. *International Journal for Philosophy of Religion, 15*(1), 89–92. https://www.ngumc.org/files/fileslibrary/james+fowlers+stages+of+faith.pdf

Francis, L., DePriest, K., Wilson, M., & Gross, D. (2018). Child poverty, toxic stress, and social determinants of health: Screening and care coordination. *Online Journal of Issues of Nursing, 23*(3). https://doi.org/10.3912/OJIN.Vol23No03Man02

Frankenburg, W., & Dodds, J. (1967). The Denver developmental screening test. *Journal of Pediatrics, 71*(2), 181–191. https://doi.org/10.1016/s0022-3476(67)80070-2

Frankenburg, W. K., Dodds, J., Archer, P., Shapiro, H., & Bresnick, B. (1992). The Denver II: A major revision and restandardization of the Denver Developmental Screening Test. *Pediatrics, 89*(1), 91–97. https://pubmed.ncbi.nlm.nih.gov/1370185/

Gardner, H. (1993). *Frames of the mind: The theory of multiple intelligences* (2nd ed.). Basic Books.

Gaufin, T., Tobin, N. H., & Aldrovandi, G. M. (2018). The importance of the microbiome in pediatrics and pediatric infectious diseases. *Current Opinion in Pediatrics, 30*(1), 117–124. https://doi.org/10.1097/MOP.0000000000000576

Girod, C., Barris, K. & Vargas, J. A. (2021). The storytellers. In A. Plough (Ed.), *Community resilience: Equitable practices for an uncertain future* (pp. 9–15). Oxford University Press.

Gitterman, B. A., Flanagan, P. J., Cotton, W. H., Dilley, K. J., Duffee, J. H., Green, A. E., Keane, V. A., Krugman, S. D., Linton, J. M., McKelvey, C. D., & Nelson, J. L. (2016). *Poverty and child health in the United States. Pediatrics, 137*(4), Article e20160339. https://doi.org/10.1542/peds.2016-0339

Gratale, D., & Haushalter, A. (2016). *Optimizing health outcomes for children with asthma in Delaware: A population health case report.* National Academy of Medicine. https://doi.org/10.31478/201609a

Groseclose, S. L., & Buckeridge, D. L. (2017). Public health surveillance systems: Recent advances in their use and evaluation. *Annual Review of Public Health, 38*, 57–79. https://doi.org/10.1146/annurev-publhealth-031816-044348

Health Resources and Services Administration. (2022, September). *The maternal, infant, and early childhood home visiting program*. https://mchb.hrsa.gov/sites/default/files/mchb/about-us/program-brief.pdf

Heisler, M., Lapidos, A., Kieffer, E., Henderson, J., Guzman, R., Cunmulaj, J., Wolfe, J., Meyer, T. & Ayanian, J. A. (2022). Impact on healthcare utilization and costs of a Medicaid community health worker program in Detroit 2018–2020: A randomized program evaluation. *American Journal of Public Health, 112*(5), 766–775. https://doi.org/10.2105/AJPH.2021.306700

Holmes, A. V., McLeod, A. Y., & Bunik, M. (2013). ABM clinical protocol #5: Peripartum breastfeeding management for the healthy mother and infant at term, revision 2013. *Breastfeeding Medicine, 8*(6), 469–473. https://doi.org/10.1089/bfm.2015.0134

Hosseini Shokouh, S. M., Arab, M., Emamgholipour, S., Rashidian, A., Montazeri, A., & Zaboli, R. (2016). Conceptual models of social determinants of health: A narrative review. *Iran Journal of Public Health, 46*(4), 435–446. http://ijph.tums.ac.ir

Institute for Functional Medicine. (n.d.). *Functional medicine determines how and why illness occurs and restores health by addressing the root causes of disease for each individual.* https://www.ifm.org/functional-%20%20%20medicine/

Institute of Medicine (US) Roundtable on Evidence-Based Medicine (2010); Yong P.L., Saunders R., S., Olsen L., A, editors. Washington (DC): National Academies Press (US).

Institute for Work and Health. (2015, April). *Primary, secondary, and tertiary prevention*. https://www.iwh.on.ca/what-researchers-mean-by/primary-secondary-and-tertiary-prevention

Iowa Department of Health and Human Services. (n.d.). *1st five: Primary care providers*. https://hhs.iowa.gov/1stfive/professionals

Johnson, K. (2017, September 30). Healthy and ready to learn: School nurses improve equity and access. *The Online Journal of Issues in Nursing, 22*(3). https://doi.org/10.3912/OJIN.Vol22No03Man01

Juvenile Diabetes Research Foundation. (n.d.). *Home*. https://www.jdrf.org

Kepper, M. M., Myers, C. A., Denstel, K. D., Hunter, R. F., Guan, W., & Broyles, S. T. (2019). The neighborhood social environment and physical activity: A systematic scoping review. *International Journal of Behavioral Nutrition and Physical Activity, 16*, Article 124. https://doi.org/10.1186/s12966-019-0873-7

Kindig D. A. (2007). Understanding population health terminology. *The Milbank quarterly, 85*(1), 139–161. https://doi.org/10.1111/j.1468-0009.2007.00479.x

Kindig, D., & Stoddart, G. (2003). What is population health? *American Journal of Public Health, 93*(3), 380–383. https://doi.org/10.2105/AJPH.93.3.380

Klaucke, D., Buehler, J., Thacker, S., Parrish, R., Trowbridge, F., & Berkelman, R. (1988). Guidelines for evaluating surveillance systems. *Centers for Disease Control and Prevention, 37*(Suppl. 5), 1–18. https://www.cdc.gov/mmwr/preview/mmwrhtml/00001769.htm

Lauwers, J., & Swisher, A. (2016). *Counseling the nursing mother: A lactation consultant's guide* (6th ed.). Jones & Bartlett Learning. Life Course Intervention Research Network. https://lcirn.ucla.edu

Makelarski, J. A., Abramsohn, E., Benjamin, J. H., Du. S., & Tessler Lindau, S. (2017). Diagnostic accuracy of two food insecurity screeners recommended for use in healthcare settings. *American Journal of Public Health, 107*(11), 1812–1817. https://doi.org/10.2105/AJPH.2017.304033

March of Dimes. (n.d.). *March for babies: A mother of a movement.* https://www.marchforbabies.org/Registration/ads-signup?utm_source=google&utm_medium=cpc&utm_campaign=2023mfb&utm_content=brand&bt=google&gclid=CjwKCAiAu5agBhBzEiwAdiR5tFZYZFPE6y1wGxTLqT4VpUrzGVAgyKhc4ksMCsYRRbN3EHqtvPv-mhoCgq4QAvD_BwE&gclsrc=aw.ds

Maughan, E. D., Bobo, N., Butler, S., & Schantz, S. (2016). Framework for 21st century school nursing practice: National Association of School Nurses. *NASN School Nurse, 31*(1), 45–53. https://doi.org/10.1177/1942602X15618644

McDermott-Levy, R., Jackman-Murphy, K. P., Leffers, J., & Cantù, A. D. (2022). *Environmental health in nursing* (2nd ed.). Alliance of Nurses for Healthy Environments. https://rfinfo.co.uk/wp-content/uploads/2022/05/Wireless-and-Non-Ionizing-EMF-Pollution-Environ-Health-in-Nursing-Dodd-Scarato-2022.pdf

McLeod, S. (2023a, March 8). *Kohlberg's stages of moral development.* Simply Psychology. https://www.simplypsychology.org/kohlberg.html#preconventional-morality

McLeod, S. A. (2023b, March 8). *Mary Ainsworth: Strange situation experiment & attachment theory.* Simply Psychology. www.simplypsychology.org/mary-ainsworth.html

Mind Help. (n.d.). *Attachment.* https://mind.help/topic/attachments/

Moretti, M. M., & Peled, M. (2004). Adolescent-parent attachment: Bonds that support healthy development. *Paediatrics & Child Health, 9*(8), 551–555. https://doi.org/10.1093/pch/9.8.551

Morone, J. (2017). An integrative review of social determinants of health assessment and screening tool used in pediatrics. *Journal of Pediatric Nursing, 37,* 22–28. https://doi.org/10.1016/j.pedn.2017.08.022

Mount Sinai. (n.d.). *Mount Sinai Adolescent Health Center.* https://www.mountsinai.org/locations/adolescent-health-center

Myers, P. (2022, November 11). *Reflecting on two decades of progress in environmental health and science communication.* Environmental Health News. https://www.ehn.org/environmental-health-and-science-communication-2658582141.html?vgo_ee=YdMxxrHqbfO41ccV%2FmDRuovy7T5YEJ8ohjC9vauJg30%3D

National Academies of Sciences, Engineering, and Medicine. (2017). *Communities in action: Pathways to health equity.* National Academies Press. https://www.ncbi.nlm.nih.gov/books/NBK425859/

National Academies of Sciences, Engineering, and Medicine. (2019). *Achieving behavioral health equity for children, families, and communities: Proceedings of a workshop.* The National Academies Press. https://doi.org/10.17226/25347.

National Academies of Sciences, Engineering, and Medicine. (2021). *The future of nursing 2020–2030: Charting a path to achieve health equity.* The National Academies Press. https://doi.org/10.17226/25982.

National Association of School Nurses. (2018, January). *Healthy communities.* https://www.nasn.org/nasn-resources/professional-practice-documents/position-statements/ps-healthy-communities

National Environmental Education Foundation Environmental. (n.d.). *Pediatric asthma.* https://www.neefusa.org/health/asthma

National Healthcare for the Homeless Council. (2019, February). *Homelessness and health: What's the connection?* https://nhchc.org/wp-content/uploads/2019/08/homelessness-and-health.pdf

Nationwide Children's. (n.d.). *The Collaboratory for kids and community health.* https://www.nationwidechildrens.org/about-us/collaboratory

New York State Department of Health. (n.d.). *Making New York the healthiest state: Achieving the triple aim*. https://www.health.ny.gov/events/population_health_summit/docs/what_is_population_health.pdf

Nsubuga, P., White, M. E., Thacker, S. B., Anderson, M. A., Blount, S. B., Broome, C. V., Chiller, T. M, Espitia, V., Imtiaz, R., Sosin, D., Stroup, D. F., Tauxe, R. V., Vijayaraghavan, M., & Trostle, M. (2006). Public health surveillance: A tool for targeting and monitoring interventions. In D. T. Jamison, J. G. Breman, A. R. Measham, G. Alleyne, M. Claeson, D. B. Evans, P. Jha, A. Mills, & P. Musgrove (Eds.), *Disease control priorities in developing countries* (2nd ed.). The World Bank. https://www.ncbi.nlm.nih.gov/books/NBK11770/

Occupational Safety and Health Administration. (n.d.). *Worker exposure risk to COVID-19*. https://www.osha.gov/sites/default/files/publications/OSHA3993.pdf

Office of Disease Prevention and Health Promotion. (n.d.-a) *Health literacy in healthy people 2030*. https://health.gov/healthypeople/priority-areas/health-literacy-healthy-people-2030

Office of Disease Prevention and Health Promotion. (n.d.-b). *Social determinants of health*. https://health.gov/healthypeople/priority-areas/social-determinants-health

Office of Disease Prevention and Health Promotion. (2022, November 14). *Newly released: Vital and health statistics series report on health disparities in healthy people 2020*. https://health.gov/news/202211/newly-released-vital-and-health-statistics-series-report-health-disparities-healthy-people-2020?source=govdelivery&utm_medium=email&utm_source=govdelivery

Pachter, L. M., Lieberman, L., Bloom, S. L., & Fein, J. A. (2017). Developing a community-wide initiative to address childhood adversity and toxic stress: A case study of the Philadelphia ACE task force. *Academic Pediatrics, 17*(7), S130–S135. http://doi.org/10.1016/j.acap.2017.04.012

Plough, A., Miller, C., & Tait, M. (2018). *Moving forward together: An update on building and measuring a culture of health*. Robert Wood Johnson Foundation. https://phinstitute.wpenginepowered.com/wp-content/uploads/2020/01/l8n8zr0qotb81905f50zruss5oh9em9y6s4pqauyddqulsm290.pdf

Pregnancy, Birth, and Baby. (n.d.). *Your baby's growth and development: 2 months old*. Australian Government Department of Health and Aged Care. https://www.pregnancybirthbaby.org.au/babys-growth-and-development-2-months-old

Public Health Institute PHI Impacts 2020 (2020). PHI Impacts 2020 - Public Health Institute

Quizhpi, C., Schetzina, K., Jaishankar, G., Tolliver, R. M., Thibeault, D., Kwak, H. G., Fapo, O., Gibson, J., Duvall, K., & Wood, D. (2019). Breaking the cycle of childhood adversity through pediatric primary care screening and interventions: A pilot study. *International Journal of Child Health & Human Development, 12*(4), 345–354. https://novapublishers.com/shop/international-journal-of-child-health-and-human-development/

Ranniger, G. (2020, June 01). *Environmental injustice*. Environmental Health News. https://www.ehn.org/environmental-justice-2646185608.html

Rees C. (2007). Childhood attachment. The British journal of general practice: the journal of the Royal College of General Practitioners, 57(544), 920–922. https://doi.org/10.3399/096016407782317955 Read more here: https://mind.help/topic/attachments/

Robert Wood Johnson Foundation. (n.d.-a). *Building a culture of health for America*. https://www.rwjf.org/en/robert-wood-johnson-foundation.html

Robert Wood Johnson Foundation. (n.d.-b). *Culture of health blog*. https://www.rwjf.org/en/insights/blog.html?o=0&us=1

Robert Wood Johnson Foundation. (n.d.-c). *Why build a culture of health*. https://www.rwjf.org/en/cultureofhealth/about/why-equity-matters.html

Robert Wood Johnson Foundation. (2018, May). *Moving forward together: An update on building and measuring a culture of health*. https://www.rwjf.org/en/library/research/2018/05/moving-foward-together--an-update-on-building-and-measuring-a-culture-of-health.html

Robert Wood Johnson Foundation. (2022, September 14). *States recognized for Medicaid program Innovations: Six states honored by RWJF and the National Academy for State Health Policy with 2022 Medicaid Innovation Award*. https://www.rwjf.org/en/about-rwjf/newsroom/2022/08/states-recognized-for-medicaid-program-innovations.html

Safekids Worlwide, (2023). Safety Tips. https://www.safekids.org/safetytips?page=6

Schickedanz,A., & Halfon, N. (2020). *Evolving Roles for Health Care in Supporting Healthy Child Development Future Child*, 30(2), 143–164.

Sharon, G., Sampson, T. R., Geschwind, D. H., & Mazmanian, S. K. (2016). The central nervous system and the gut microbiome. *Cell, 167*(4), 915–932. https://doi.org/10.1016/j.cell.2016.10.027

Shrank, W. H., Rogstad, T. L., & Parekh, N. (2019). Waste in the U.S. healthcare system: Estimated costs and potential or savings. *JAMA, 322*(15), 1501–1509. https://doi.org/10.1001/jama.2019.13978

Shreiner, A. B., Kao, J. Y., & Young, V. B. (2015). The gut microbiome in health and in disease. *Current Opinion in Gastroenterology, 31*(1), 69–75. https://doi.org/10.1097/MOG.0000000000000139

Slykerman, R. F., Thompson, J., Waldie, K. E., Murphy, R., Wall, C., & Mitchell, E. A. (2017). Antibiotics in the first year of life and subsequent neurocognitive outcomes. *Acta Paediatrica, 106*(1), 87–94. https://doi.org/10.1111/apa.13613

Sokol , R., Austin , A. Chandler , C., Byrum , E., Bousquette , J., Lancaster 2, C., Doss , G., Dotson, A., Urbaeva, V., Singichetti , B., Brevard , B., Towner Wright , S., Lanier, P., Shanahan, M. (2019). Screening children for the social determinates of health. *Pediatrics, 144*(4):e20191622. doi: 10.1542/peds.2019-1622

Stiemsma L. T., & Michels, K. B. (2018). The role of the microbiome in the developmental origins of health and disease. *Pediatrics, 141*(4), Article e20172437. https://doi.org/10.1542/peds.2017-2437

Swartout M., & Bishop, M. (2017). *Different scholars define population health*. Course Hero. https://www.coursehero.com/file/77261520/Different-scholars-define-population-health-differentlydocx/

Teitelbaum, J. B., & Wilensky, S. E. (2017). *Essentials of health policy and law* (3rd ed.). Jones & Bartlett Learning.

Thomas, A., Chess, S., & Birch, H. G. (1968). *Temperament and behavior disorders in children*. New York University Press.

Thomas, F., & Fietje, N. (2020). Capturing the cultural narrative of wellbeing. In A. Plough (Ed.), *Well-being: Expanding the definition of progress* (pp. 67–82). Oxford University Press.

Thomson Delmar Learning. (2007). *Children's development*. https://www.ccmedical.org/forms/1428352937_171971.pdf

The Trevor Project. (n.d.). *Home*. https://www.thetrevorproject.org

Travis, J. (1977). *Wellness workbook for health professionals: A guide to attaining high level wellness* (1st ed.). Wellness Resource Center.

Travis, J. W. (1988). *Wellness inventory* (3rd ed.) Wellness Lifestyle.

Two Rivers Ottauquechee Regional Commission. (2020). *Two Rivers-Ottauquechee Regional Plan*. https://www.trorc.org/wp-content/uploads/2020/09/TRORC2020RegionalPlan_finalMOBmaps.pdf

Uchima, O., Sentell, T., Dela Cruz, R. M., & Braun, K. L. (2019). Community health workers in pediatric asthma education programs in the United States: A systematic literature review. *Children's Healthcare, 48*(2), 215–243. https://doi.org/10.1080/02739615.2018.1520107

University of Wisconsin Population Health Institute. (n.d.). *County health rankings and roadmaps*. https://www.countyhealthrankings.org/

U.S. Census Bureau. (2021, August 12). *Racial and ethnic diversity in the United States: 2010 census and 2020 census*. https://www.census.gov/library/visualizations/interactive/racial-and-ethnic-diversity-in-the-united-states-2010-and-2020-census.html

U.S. Department of Health and Human Services. (n.d.-a). *Find a Health Center* [Map]. Health Resources and Services Administration Data Warehouse. https://findahealthcenter.hrsa.gov

U.S. Department of Health and Human Services. (n.d.-b). *Head start center locater* [Map]. Head Start and Early Head Start. https://eclkc.ohs.acf.hhs.gov/center-locator

Valdes, A. M., Walter, J., Segal, E., Spector, T. D. (2018). Role of the gut microbiota in nutrition and health. *BMJ, 361*, 36–44. https://doi.org/10.1136/bmj.k2179

Walker, G. C., Martinez-Gómez, V., & Gonzalez, R. O. (2018, September 30). Mobile traveling healthcare teams: An innovative delivery system for underserved populations. *The Online Journal of Issues in Nursing, 23*(3). https://doi.org/10.3912/OJIN.Vol23No03Man03

Wang, L. Y., Vernon-Smiley, M., Gapinski, M. A., Desisto, M., Maughan, E., & Sheetz, A. (2014). Cost-benefit study of school nursing services. *JAMA Pediatrics, 168*(7), 642–648. https://doi.org/10.1001/jamapediatrics.2013.5441

Ward, S., & Hisley, S. (2016). *Maternal child nursing care: Optimizing outcomes for mothers, children and families* (2nd ed.). FA Davis.

Weinstein, J. N., Geller, A., Negussie, Y., & Baciu, A. (2017). *Communities in action: Pathways to health equity.* National Academy of Sciences. https://www.ncbi.nlm.nih.gov/books/NBK425848/pdf/Bookshelf_NBK425848.pdf

White-Means, S., Gaskin, D. J., & Osmani, A. R. (2019). Intervention and public policy pathways to achieve healthcare equity. *International Journal of Environmental Research and Public Health, 16*(14), Article 2465. https://doi.org/10.3390/ijerph16142465

Wickramarathne, P., Phuoc, J., & Albattat, A. (2020). A review of wellness dimension models: For the advancement of the society. *European Journal of Social Sciences Studies, 5*(1). https://doi.org/10.5281/zenodo.3841435

Widström, A. M., Brimdyr, K., Svensson, K., Cadwell, K., & Nissen, E. (2019), Skin-to-skin contact the first hour after birth, underlying implications and clinical practice. *Acta Paediatrica, 108*(7), 1192–1204. https://doi.org/10.1111/apa.14754

Williams, S. D., Phillips, J. M., & Koyama, K. (2018, September 30). Nurse advocacy: Adopting a health in all policies approach. *The Online Journal of Issues in Nursing, 23*(3). https://doi.org/10.3912/OJIN.Vol23No03Man01

Wilson AL, Jovanovic JM, Harman-Smith YE, Ward PR. (2019). A population health approach in education to support children's early development: A Critical Interpretive Synthesis. *PLOS One, 14*(6):e0218403. doi: 10.1371/journal.pone.0218403. PMID: 31199851; PMCID: PMC6568401.

World Health Organization. (n.d.). *About us.* https://www.emro.who.int/about-who/public-health-functions/health-promotion-disease-prevention.html

World Health Organization. (2016, August 20). *Health promotion.* https://www.who.int/news-room/questions-and-answers/item/health-promotion

Wyatt, R. (2016). *What's the relationship between health equity and the triple aim?* Institute for Healthcare Improvement. https://www.ihi.org/Engage/Initiatives/TripleAim/Pages/default.aspx

YWCA. (n.d.). *Understanding the history and mission of the YWCA.* https://www.ywcatricountyarea.org/who-we-are/

INDEX

ABOUT THE AUTHORS

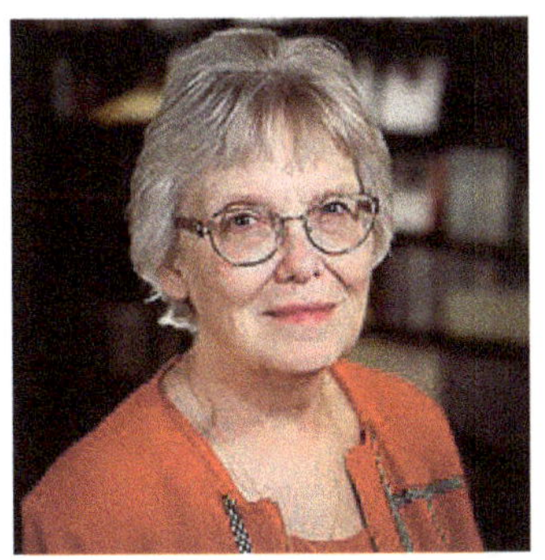
Image 0.1

Dr. Susan Ward's desire to help others came at an early age when she was a Methodist Hospital candy striper. That is when she discovered a lifelong passion for nursing. She has been a registered nurse (RN) since 1979. Dr. Ward earned an associate degree in nursing (1979-University of Nebraska); bachelor's degree in nursing (1980-University of Nebraska Medical Center); master's degree in nursing (1990-University of Nebraska Medical Center); and Ph.D. in adult education/community and community and human resources (2000-University of Nebraska).

Dr. Ward has published several books, as well as journal and research articles spanning from 1997 to 2023. She is the co-author of *Maternal Child Nursing Care: Optimizing Outcomes for Mothers, Children, and Families*, which received two American Journal of Nursing Awards. Examples of other works published include: *Faith Community Nursing: Scope and Standards of Practice* (American Nurses Association); *Pediatric Nursing Care: Best Evidence-Based Practices*; Collaborative Student Leadership Conference; *Accelerated Nursing Education: The New Careers in Nursing Scholarship Program - Innovations and Legacy*; *Journal of Professional Nursing*; and qualitative data analysis for "Women's Experience with Celiac Disease: A Phenomenological Study," *Gastroenterology Nurses and Associates*.

Her podium and poster presentations on a local, state, regional, and national levels are also numerous. Additional involvement in professional nursing includes membership in the Nebraska Nurses Association and National League for Nursing; chair of the AANC Practice Ready Group for Competency-Based Education for Practice-Ready Nurse Graduates; assisted writing the Veterans Administration and Methodist Health System Nurse Residency programs; member of the COVID-19 Scarce Resource Team and Covid-19 Committee Response committee; Iowa Western Community College Nursing Advisory Board; and article reviewer for the *Journal for Specialists in Pediatric Nursing* and *Journal of Professional Nursing*. She has also written and received numerous grants, including the AACN and Robert Wood Johnson Foundation New Careers in Nursing grant, and volunteers for the Linus Project.

Dr. Ward has 44 years of nursing practice and nursing education. Her post-secondary educational experience included several years of leadership, teaching, course development, and coordination in both undergraduate and graduate programs for in-person, hybrid, and online courses. In the development of a new BSN curriculum at Nebraska Methodist College, Dr. Ward led a team of experienced nurse educators to design, implement, and evaluate a new population health curriculum that began in Fall 2020 at Nebraska Methodist College.

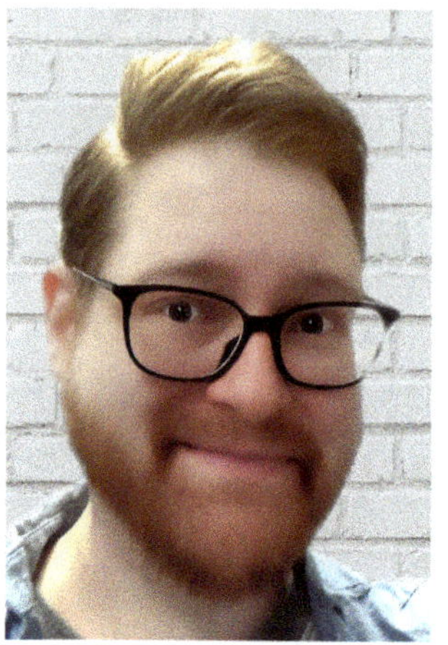

Frankie Ward earned a BA from the University of East Anglia, Norwich England and has an MS in physiology and biomechanics, MA in English, and MFA in creative nonfiction. He completed his graduate fellowship at Trinity Laban Conservatoire of Music and Dance, London in the Dance Sciences Department. Additionally, he has received apprenticeships and fellowships in writing from Metropolitan Community College and the University of Nebraska at Omaha. He is an instructor of English at the University of Nebraska at Omaha, an instructor of humanities at Nebraska Methodist College, and a Writing Center consultant at Metropolitan Community College.

ABOUT THE CONTRIBUTORS

Alice Kindschuh

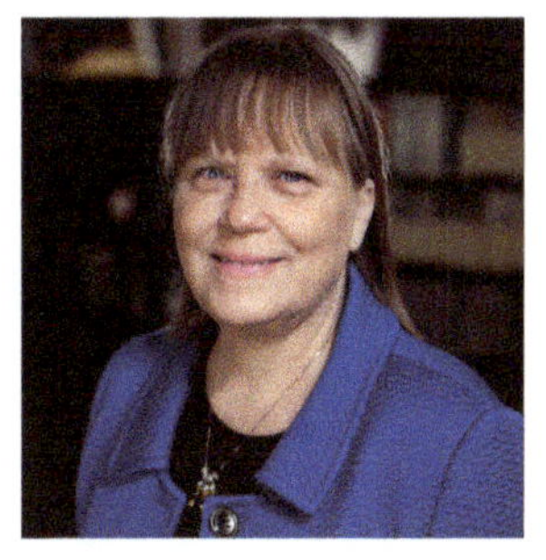
Image 0.3

Dr. Alice Kindschuh serves as the director of Doctoral Studies at Nebraska Methodist College. During her vast nursing career, Dr. Kindschuh has been instrumental in creating, teaching, and evaluating population health material and has led many conversations and initiatives for audiences on the local, state, regional and national levels. Other areas of her distinct influence are health policy, health systems, rural health, community program planning, and conducting collaborative population health efforts in the broader community. Dr. Kindschuh is highly respected among her peers as an educator, innovator, motivator and, overall, an outstanding nurse leader.

Kiley Petersmith

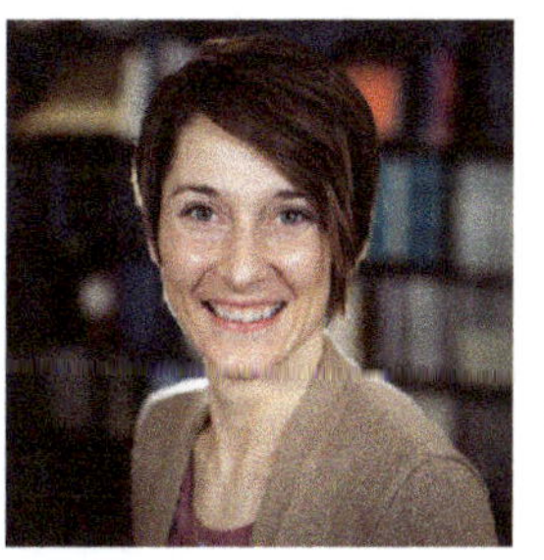
Image 0.4

Dr. Kiley Petersmith serves as the director of Diversity and Community Engagement at Nebraska Methodist College. During her nursing career, she worked in pediatrics as a critical care and emergency department nurse. She is adept at building relationships and directing the strategic visions of community engagement. Dr. Petersmith shapes meaningful and mutually beneficial community engagement experiences to address diverse community needs, creating positive social change toward equitable health and cultivating active citizen leaders. Dr. Petersmith's population health efforts emphasize prevention and the eradication of health disparities based on race, ethnicity, language, income, gender, sexual orientation, and disability.

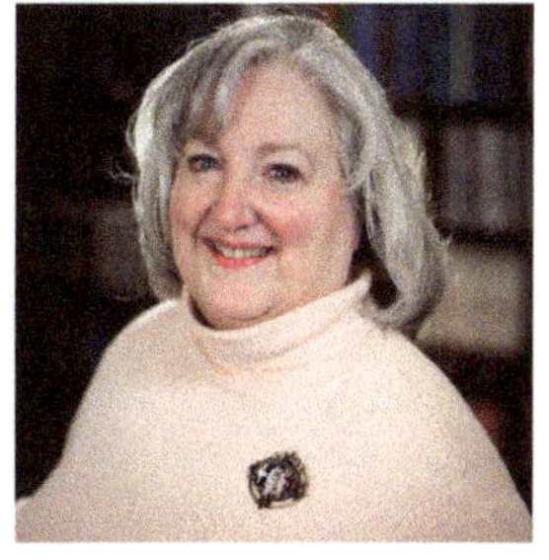
Image 0.5

Meg Blair

Dr. Meg Blair has been a nurse educator since 1995 and has extensive experience teaching and leading courses at all levels of BSN education. Throughout her career in nursing education, she has been recognized for innovative teaching methodologies, unique active learning strategies, and test-writing expertise. Currently serving as the testing specialist at Nebraska Methodist College, Dr. Blair works with both BSN faculty and students in test-writing and test-taking skills. Dr. Blair has authored over 30 test banks to accompany textbooks, multiple articles, book chapters, and coauthored a popular nursing textbook. Dr. Blair is a respected faculty member and nurse leader at Nebraska Methodist College and in the broader health care community.

Credits

www.ingramcontent.com/pod-product-compliance
Ingram Content Group UK Ltd.
Pitfield, Milton Keynes, MK11 3LW, UK
UKHW050141280726
14058UKWH00006B/761

9 798823 306713